YOGA FOR HEALTHY KNEES

My Personal Journey and Your Path to Wellness

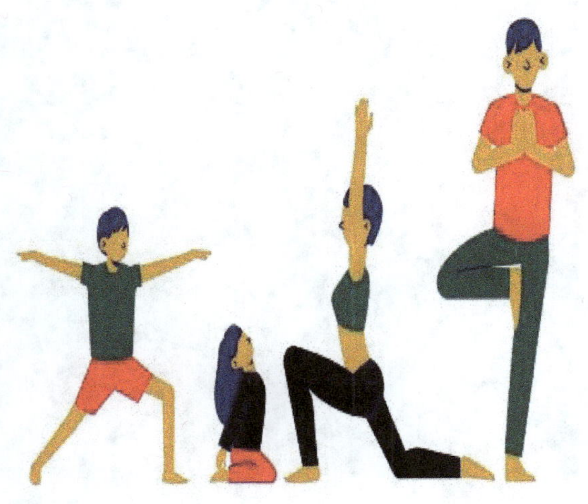

Maxwell Fitwell

TABLE OF CONTENT

INTRODUCTION

In the quiet embrace of my yoga mat, I discovered a profound transformation, one that extended far beyond the mat itself. This is a story of how I mended not just my knees but my entire life, one gentle stretch at a time.

I am Maxwell, a name I once associated with discomfort, instability, and fear due to persistent knee issues. Each step I took was a reminder of my fragility. The burden of pain dictated my choices and dreams. Yet, the universe had a different plan for me – it unfolded in the form of yoga.

As I dipped my toes into the world of yoga, I was met with skepticism. Could gentle movements, deep breaths, and the meditative stillness of yoga really be the elixir my knees needed? Little did I know that this ancient practice held the power to mend not only my knees but also my mind, body, and soul.

Yoga became my sanctuary, a place where I could heal, grow, and thrive. With each asana, I nurtured not just the physical strength in my knees but the inner resilience that had long eluded me. The slow, deliberate sequences allowed me to listen to my body, to understand its needs, and to move in harmony with it.

Through my journey, I uncovered a world of invaluable wisdom and practices tailored specifically to those seeking knee health and overall well-being. My commitment to my practice and the remarkable benefits I reaped along the way became the inspiration for this book – "Yoga for Healthy Knees."

This book is my gift to you, my fellow seekers of vitality and strength. It's a carefully crafted roadmap, born out of my own struggles, failures, and ultimate triumphs. It's the bridge between your dreams of pain-free, agile knees and the reality of living that life. Inside, you'll find not only the postures and techniques that transformed my knees but also the mental and emotional shifts that allowed me to regain control of my life.

"Yoga for Healthy Knees" is a testament to the power of this ancient practice to heal, strengthen, and transform. It's a promise that your journey can be as rewarding and enlightening as mine. So, dear reader, whether you're facing knee troubles or simply seeking a holistic approach to health and well-being, I invite you to step onto the path of healing and transformation with me. Let's begin this transformative journey together, one breath, one stretch, and one chapter at a time.

Welcome to Yoga for Healthy Knees: A Journey to Pain-Free Mobility and Inner Well-Being

In the hustle and bustle of our daily lives, it's easy to take the simple act of walking for granted. Yet, for those who have experienced the discomfort, pain, and limitations that knee issues can bring, each step can feel like a triumph. If you've ever wrestled with knee pain, instability, or discomfort, you're not alone. Millions of individuals around the world share your struggles, and like them, you've probably explored countless avenues searching for relief.

But today, you've taken a significant step forward on your path to healing, strength, and well-being. Welcome to "Yoga for Healthy Knees," a comprehensive guide that promises to be your compass on this transformative journey.

This isn't just another yoga book; it's your passport to pain-free mobility and inner peace. Through the pages of this guide, you'll embark on a profound exploration of how the ancient practice of yoga can be a potent elixir for your knee health and your overall quality of life.

What Awaits You in These Pages

1. The Power of Yoga for Knee Health: We'll delve into the science behind yoga and its remarkable ability to strengthen and heal your knees. You'll discover how gentle movements and stretches can alleviate pain, improve flexibility, and enhance stability.

2. Personal Stories of Transformation: Throughout this book, you'll encounter inspiring stories from individuals who, like you, embarked on their yoga journey to healthier knees. You'll find solace in knowing that others have faced similar challenges and found success through yoga.

3. A Holistic Approach to Well-Being: "Yoga for Healthy Knees" goes beyond the physical. We'll explore how yoga's mental and emotional facets can empower you to take control of your life, manage stress, and embrace a newfound sense of balance.

4. Detailed Postures and Sequences: You'll find a treasure trove of yoga postures specifically curated to alleviate knee pain and promote strength. Whether you're a seasoned yogi or just starting, our step-by-step instructions will guide you.

5. Mindful Breathing and Meditation Practices: Learn to harness the incredible power of your breath and unlock the potential of meditation for stress reduction, mental clarity, and overall well-being.

6. Tailored Routines for Your Needs: We understand that no two knees are the same. You'll discover routines designed for various levels, from gentle beginners' sequences to advanced practices, allowing you to choose what suits you best.

7. Expert Advice and Tips: Benefit from expert insights, tips, and precautions to ensure that your yoga practice is safe, effective, and tailored to your unique needs.

8. Building a Lifelong Practice: Our goal is not just to help you find relief; it's to equip you with the tools and knowledge to make yoga a lifelong companion for your knee health and overall well-being.

9. Your Personal Journey: "Yoga for Healthy Knees" is more than a book; it's an invitation to transform your life. As you embark on this journey, you'll realize that you are not just mending your knees; you're rediscovering the boundless potential within yourself.

So, welcome to a world of possibilities, dear reader. It is time to begin a journey of self-discovery, healing, and change. "Yoga for Healthy Knees" is your trusted companion on this journey, guiding you toward a future where every step you take is a step toward vitality, strength, and inner well-being.

The adventure begins here. Let's take that first step together.

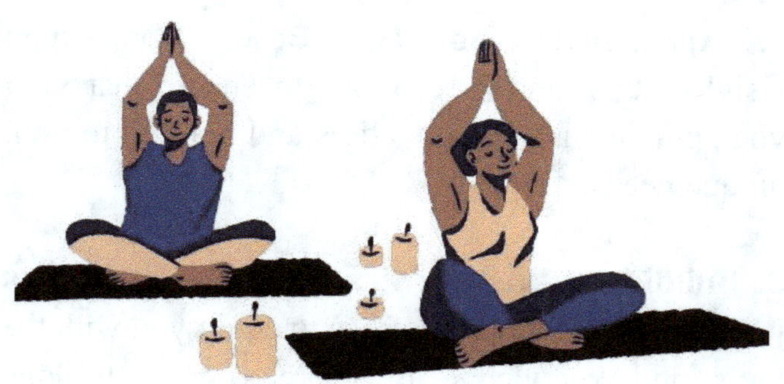

Why Yoga for Knee Health?

Your knees are incredible joints, enabling you to walk, run, dance, and move through life's adventures. However, when knee pain and discomfort strike, they can become an unwelcome obstacle in your journey. This is where the magic of yoga comes into play. Let's explore why yoga is your perfect ally for achieving and maintaining optimal knee health.

1. Gentle, Targeted Healing:
Yoga offers a gentle and effective way to heal your knees. Its low-impact, controlled movements and stretches can alleviate pain, improve flexibility, and enhance stability. Unlike high-impact exercises, which can exacerbate knee issues, yoga nurtures your knees with care.

2. Holistic Approach:
Yoga isn't just about physical postures. It encompasses a holistic approach that addresses both the physical and mental aspects of well-being. It's not merely about strengthening your knees; it's about nurturing your overall health and vitality.

3. Mind-Body Connection:
Yoga's emphasis on the mind-body connection is one of its most notable features. Through yoga,

you'll learn to listen to your body, understand its needs, and move in harmony with it. This deep awareness empowers you to make choices that promote knee health and pain-free living.

4. Stress Reduction:

Stress is often a contributing factor to knee pain. The meditative aspects of yoga, including mindful breathing and meditation, can reduce stress and provide you with mental clarity and emotional balance. When your mind is at ease, your knees tend to follow suit.

5. Customized for You:

Yoga is incredibly versatile, and practices can be tailored to your unique needs. Whether you're a beginner or an experienced yogi, you can find postures and routines that suit your current level of fitness and flexibility. This adaptability ensures that yoga is accessible to virtually anyone.

6. Long-Term Solutions:

Yoga doesn't offer quick fixes; it's a long-term solution for knee health. By consistently practicing yoga, you can build strength, flexibility, and resilience in your knees, reducing the risk of future issues and maintaining your mobility as you age.

7. Supportive Community:

Yoga often comes with a built-in community of like-minded individuals. Sharing your journey with others who are also working toward knee health can be incredibly motivating and supportive. You'll find encouragement, advice, and a sense of belonging in the yoga community.

8. Expert Guidance:

In "Yoga for Healthy Knees," you'll have access to expert guidance and tips to ensure your yoga practice is safe, effective, and tailored to your needs. This book is your comprehensive resource for embarking on a journey to pain-free knees and vibrant health.

9. Beyond Knees:

While the focus of yoga for knee health is evident, the benefits extend beyond your knees. Your entire body will benefit from improved flexibility, strength, and balance. Your mind will benefit from reduced stress, increased focus, and emotional well-being.

10. Empowerment:

Yoga empowers you to be in control of your health. It's a proactive approach that allows you to actively participate in your well-being. With yoga, you're not just managing knee pain; you're on a path to thriving and living life to the fullest.

"Yoga for Knee Health" isn't just about healing; it's about transformation. It's about finding the strength within yourself to overcome knee pain and embrace a life filled with mobility, vitality, and inner well-being. So, if you're ready to embark on a journey toward healthier, pain-free knees, you've come to the right place. Welcome to the world of yoga, where your knees are not obstacles but the keys to unlocking your full potential.

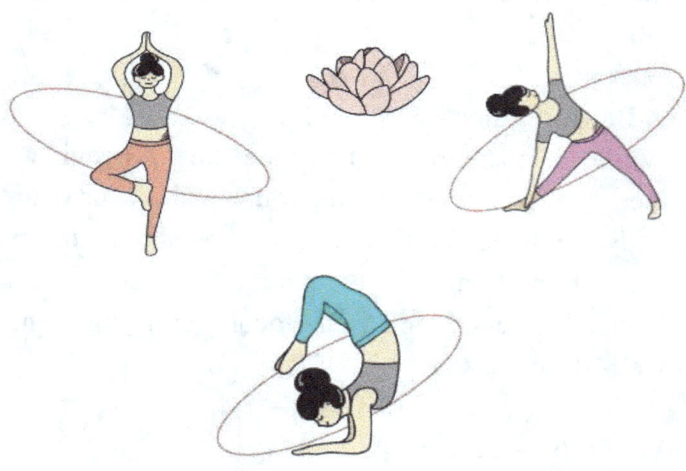

Chapter 1: Understanding Knee Health

In the intricate landscape of your body, your knees serve as pillars of strength and flexibility. To embark on the journey toward healthier knees, it's essential to first understand their intricate design, the common challenges they face, and the role yoga plays in nurturing them back to vitality. Welcome to the foundation of your path to knee health.

Anatomy of the Knee

Unlocking the Secrets of Your Body's Hinges

To truly appreciate and care for your knees, it's crucial to embark on a journey beneath the skin, to explore the intricate workings of one of the most remarkable joints in the human body. Welcome to the realm of knee anatomy, where the keys to unlocking the secrets of your body's hinges are found.

1. The Knee Joint: A Marvel of Engineering
Your knee is the biggest and one of the most complicated joints in your body. It's where the thigh bone (femur), the shin bone (tibia), and the kneecap

(patella) come together in a highly evolved hinge joint. This design allows for the incredible range of motion that enables activities from walking and running to bending and stretching.

2. Bones and Their Roles

- **Femur**: The thigh bone, which extends from your hip to your knee. It carries the body's weight and connects with the tibia to form the main hinge of the knee joint.

- **Tibia**: Also known as the *shin bone*, it extends from the knee to the ankle and bears the weight that's transferred through the knee joint.

- **Patella**: The kneecap is a sesamoid bone situated within the quadriceps tendon. It acts as a fulcrum, increasing the leverage of the quadriceps muscles, which are crucial for knee extension.

3. Articular Cartilage: Nature's Shock Absorber

Within the knee joint, the surfaces of the femur, tibia, and patella are coated with a smooth, shiny material called articular cartilage. This remarkable substance reduces friction, allowing the bones to glide effortlessly against each other. Think of it as nature's shock absorber, preventing the bones from grinding together during movement.

4. Ligaments: Stability Guardians

Ligaments are tough, fibrous bands that connect bones and provide stability to joints. In the knee, you'll find several crucial ligaments:

- **ACL (Anterior Cruciate Ligament):** Prevents the tibia from moving too far forward relative to the femur.

- **PCL (Posterior Cruciate Ligament):** Does the opposite, preventing the tibia from moving too far backward.

- **MCL (Medial Collateral Ligament) and LCL (Lateral Collateral Ligament):** These provide side-to-side stability, preventing the knee from buckling.

5. Muscles: The Dynamic Engines

The muscles surrounding the knee are responsible for its movement and stability. Notable players include:

- **Quadriceps**: These muscles on the front of the thigh extend the knee.

- **Hamstrings**: Situated on the back of the thigh, they flex the knee.

- **Calf muscles**: Found in the lower leg, they play a role in knee stability and mobility.

6. Menisci: Nature's Cushions
Imagine two wedge-shaped shock absorbers made of tough cartilage within your knee joint – those are the menisci. They enhance stability, absorb shock, and distribute the body's weight evenly across the joint.

7. Synovial Fluid: Lubrication for Smooth Movement
Inside the knee joint, synovial fluid is the lubricant that keeps everything moving smoothly. It reduces friction and nourishes the articular cartilage, ensuring your knee operates seamlessly.

8. The Fascinating Biomechanics
Understanding knee anatomy is crucial for understanding how injuries occur and why certain yoga postures and exercises are beneficial. Your knees are not just hinges; they are a marvel of engineering, a symphony of interconnected elements working in harmony to facilitate your every move.

Why Does This Matter?

By delving into the anatomy of your knees, you're not just gaining knowledge; you're equipping yourself with the understanding needed to care for them. Whether you're managing existing knee issues or striving for a future of pain-free mobility, this knowledge is your first step.

So, welcome to the world of knee anatomy. You're now armed with the foundation to explore how yoga can become your ally in nurturing, healing, and strengthening this intricate joint. With this understanding, you're ready to unlock the full potential of your knees and embark on a journey to knee health and well-being.

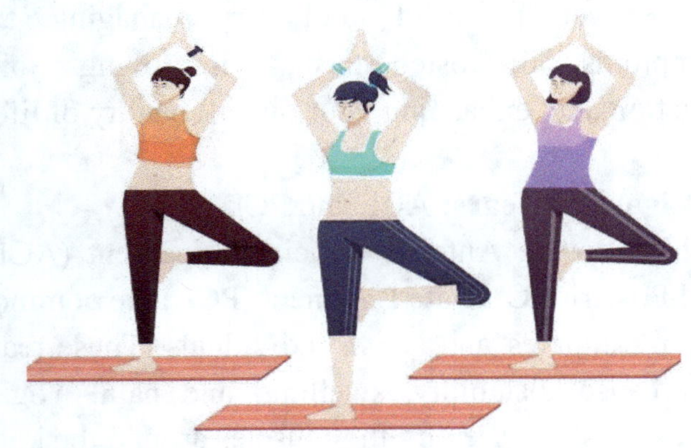

Common Knee Issues

Identifying and Conquering the Hurdles to Health

Your knees, marvels of engineering as they are, can sometimes encounter challenges that hinder your mobility and well-being. Understanding these common knee issues is the first step in addressing them effectively. Now, we will explore these hurdles and equip you with knowledge on how to overcome them.

1. Osteoarthritis: The Wear and Tear

Osteoarthritis is a prevalent knee issue, often associated with aging and overuse. It's characterized by the breakdown of articular cartilage, leading to pain, stiffness, and reduced mobility. Yoga can be a gentle yet powerful tool for managing the symptoms of osteoarthritis, improving joint function, and enhancing your overall quality of life.

2. Ligament Tears: ACL and PCL

Injuries to the Anterior Cruciate Ligament (ACL) and Posterior Cruciate Ligament (PCL) are common among athletes and active individuals. These tears can cause instability, swelling, and pain. Yoga's focus on strengthening the muscles around the knee can provide crucial support during recovery and help prevent future injuries.

3. Meniscus Tears: The Shock Absorber's Woes

Your menisci are prone to tears, often as a result of sudden twisting movements. These tears can lead to pain, swelling, and mechanical symptoms like catching or locking of the knee. Yoga's emphasis on gentle, controlled movements can aid in rehabilitating the meniscus and restoring knee function.

4. Patellofemoral Pain Syndrome: The Kneecap Conundrum

When your kneecap doesn't move smoothly in its groove, it can lead to pain around or behind the kneecap, known as patellofemoral pain syndrome. Yoga's focus on balancing muscle strength and flexibility can be a valuable strategy in addressing this issue.

5. Bursitis: The Inflammation Woe

Bursae are small sacs filled with fluid that reduce friction between tissues. When they become inflamed, it leads to bursitis, causing pain and swelling. Yoga's gentle stretches and mobility exercises can alleviate this inflammation and improve knee comfort.

6. Tendonitis: Straining the Tendons
Inflammation of the tendons surrounding the knee can cause pain and discomfort. Yoga's slow, controlled movements and stretching can aid in the healing of tendonitis while preventing further strain.

7. Overuse Injuries: A Common Culprit
Repetitive stress on the knee from activities like running or high-impact sports can lead to overuse injuries. Yoga's low-impact nature and focus on balanced strength and flexibility can be an effective preventive and rehabilitative measure.

8. Cartilage Defects: A Nurturing Approach
In some cases, defects or lesions may occur in the knee's articular cartilage, leading to pain and discomfort. Yoga, with its gentle and controlled movements, can be a supportive measure in managing these issues.

Why Does This Matter?

Understanding common knee issues is pivotal because it allows you to identify your unique challenges and tailor your approach to knee health accordingly. It's the first step in the journey to overcoming these hurdles and achieving pain-free, agile knees.

The Benefits of Yoga for Knee Health

A Path to Strength, Flexibility, and Pain Relief

Yoga, with its ancient roots and timeless wisdom, offers a treasure trove of benefits for knee health. It's a holistic approach that combines physical postures, mindful breathing, and mental clarity to nurture your knees and alleviate discomfort. Let's explore the myriad advantages of incorporating yoga into your life for the sake of your knee health.

1. Pain Relief and Management:

One of the most immediate benefits of yoga for knee health is pain relief. Gentle movements and stretches, such as those found in Hatha or Restorative yoga, can help reduce knee pain, especially in cases of conditions like osteoarthritis. Yoga's low-impact nature ensures that it doesn't exacerbate pain, making it a suitable option for those with knee discomfort.

2. Improved Range of Motion:

Yoga's focus on flexibility is instrumental in enhancing the range of motion in your knees. Regular practice encourages better joint lubrication, reducing stiffness, and allowing for smoother, more pain-free movement.

3. Strength and Stability:

The muscles around your knees play a crucial role in their stability. Yoga postures like Warrior poses and Chair pose, among others, help strengthen the quadriceps, hamstrings, and calf muscles, fortifying your knees against potential issues and improving overall stability.

4. Enhanced Alignment:

Yoga is exceptional at enhancing body awareness and alignment. By paying attention to your posture and movements, you can avoid placing unnecessary stress on your knees. This awareness can be especially valuable for those recovering from knee injuries or surgeries.

5. Weight Management:

Excess body weight can strain the knee joints, exacerbating pain and discomfort. Yoga's combination of physical activity and mindfulness can aid in weight management, which, in turn, reduces the load on your knees.

6. Mind-Body Connection:

Yoga isn't solely about physical postures; it's also a practice of the mind. The stress-reducing and calming effects of yoga can help manage emotional pain and frustration that often accompany knee issues. A serene mind contributes to overall well-being and can be a powerful tool in the healing process.

7. Customization for Your Needs:

Yoga is incredibly versatile, with practices that can be tailored to your unique requirements. Whether you're a beginner or an experienced yogi, you can find routines that fit your current level of fitness and flexibility.

8. Preventative Measures:

Yoga isn't just about addressing current knee issues; it's also a preventive measure. By incorporating yoga into your routine, you can reduce the risk of future knee problems. It's a proactive approach to ensure the longevity of your knee health.

9. Holistic Approach:

Yoga's holistic nature considers not only your physical health but also your mental and emotional well-being. A healthy mind supports a healthy body, making it an all-encompassing solution for overall wellness.

10. Community and Support:
Yoga often comes with a supportive community of fellow practitioners. Sharing your journey with others who understand your challenges can be motivating and provide you with a sense of belonging.

Yoga isn't just an exercise; it's a way of life that can transform your knee health and your overall quality of life. It's a gentle yet potent approach that combines physical and mental well-being, providing relief, strength, and resilience. So, if you're ready to experience the many benefits of yoga for knee health, you're on the right path. Welcome to a future of pain-free knees, mobility, and inner well-being.

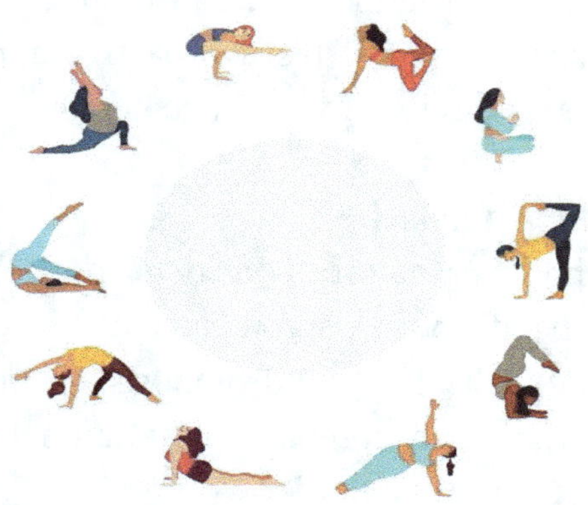

Chapter 2: Getting Started with Yoga

In the pages of this chapter, we embark on an exciting journey. It's the beginning of your exploration of yoga, a practice that will not only transform your knee health but also your overall well-being. Let's dive into the foundations, the essential tools, and the mindset required to make yoga an integral part of your life. Welcome to the threshold of a healthier, more vibrant you.

Essentials for Your Yoga Practice

Building the Foundation of Well-Being

As you step into the world of yoga, it's essential to equip yourself with the right tools and mindset to make your practice effective and rewarding. These essentials will not only enhance your yoga experience but also play a pivotal role in your journey to healthier knees and overall well-being.

1. Yoga Mat: Your Sacred Space

A quality yoga mat is your foundation. It provides a comfortable, non-slip surface for your practice. Look for a mat that supports your joints and provides ample cushioning while ensuring a stable base for your poses.

2. Comfortable Clothing: Freedom of Movement
Choose comfortable, breathable clothing that allows freedom of movement. It should be non-restrictive and moisture-wicking to keep you cool during your practice.

3. Props: Your Support System
Yoga props such as blocks, straps, and bolsters can enhance your practice. They assist with alignment, provide support in challenging poses, and make yoga accessible for all levels. These props can be especially useful when adapting your practice to accommodate knee issues.

4. Water Bottle: Hydration on Standby
Staying hydrated is vital during your practice. Keep a water bottle nearby to sip water as needed. Proper hydration ensures your muscles and joints function optimally.

5. Quiet Space: Your Sanctuary
Choose a peaceful, clutter-free space for your practice. Whether it's a corner of a room or a serene outdoor spot, your practice space should inspire tranquility and focus.

6. Open Mind and Patience: The Mindset of Growth

Yoga is not just about physical postures; it's a mindset. Approach your practice with an open mind and patience. Be kind with yourself and accept that development may be slow. Accept the journey as a chance for personal growth.

7. Consistency: The Key to Progress

Consistency is the cornerstone of a successful yoga practice. Dedicate time regularly to your practice, even if it's just a few minutes each day. It's the cumulative effect of consistent effort that yields the most significant results.

8. Breath Awareness: Your Lifeline

Your breath is your most valuable tool in yoga. Pay attention to your breath, using it to guide your movements and promote relaxation. Learning to breathe mindfully can have a profound impact on your practice and knee health.

9. Proper Technique: Quality Over Quantity

Focus on the quality of your practice rather than quantity. It's more important to execute postures with proper technique and alignment, especially when you're working with knee issues. This approach not only reduces the risk of injury but also maximizes the benefits.

10. Guidance and Learning: The Never-ending Journey

Consider taking classes, either in-person or online, to receive guidance and expand your knowledge. Books, videos, and expert advice can be invaluable resources to deepen your understanding of yoga and its benefits.

11. Modification and Adaptation: Listen to Your Body

Learn to adapt your practice to suit your unique needs. If you have knee issues, this might mean modifying certain poses or using props for support. The ability to listen to your body and adjust your practice is a sign of wisdom and self-care.

These essentials are the building blocks of a successful and fulfilling yoga practice. They pave the way for you to embrace the transformative power of yoga not only for your knees but for your entire well-being. As you incorporate these essentials into your practice, you're forging a path toward vitality, strength, and inner peace.

Preparing Your Space

Crafting a Sanctuary for Your Practice

The space in which you practice yoga is not just a physical location; it's a sanctuary for your mind, body, and soul. Preparing this space thoughtfully can significantly enhance the effectiveness and enjoyment of your practice. Here's how to create the ideal environment for your yoga journey:

1. Clutter-Free Zone: A Clear Canvas

Start by decluttering your practice area. Remove any unnecessary items that might distract you or create a sense of chaos. A clear, open space is like a blank canvas for your practice, allowing you to focus solely on your yoga journey.

2. Natural Light: Embrace the Elements

Whenever possible, choose a space with natural light. Sunlight can uplift your mood and add a calming, natural element to your practice. If natural light isn't an option, consider soft, warm artificial lighting to create a serene atmosphere.

3. Peace and Quiet: Your Inner Sanctum

Choose a location that is quiet and peaceful. Minimize external distractions by selecting a place where you won't be interrupted. Peaceful surroundings will help you connect more deeply with your practice.

4. Yoga Mat Placement: Your Sacred Ground
Your yoga mat is your sacred ground, so choose its placement carefully. Ensure it's centered in your space, with enough room around it for movement. Your mat should symbolize the boundary between your inner world and the external environment.

5. Props and Accessories: Within Reach
If you use yoga props such as blocks, straps, or bolsters, have them nearby for easy access. This ensures that your practice flows seamlessly, without interruptions to fetch the tools you need.

6. Personal Touch: Inspirational Elements
Add elements that inspire and soothe you. It might be a small altar with candles, incense, or a few cherished objects. These personal touches can create a tranquil atmosphere and serve as a reminder of the purpose of your practice.

7. Comfortable Temperature: Balance is Key
Maintain a comfortable temperature in your practice area. You don't want to be too cold or too hot during your practice, as extreme temperatures can be distracting. Find a balance that suits you.

8. Audio Ambiance: Soothing Sounds
Consider playing soft, instrumental music or nature sounds to enhance the ambiance. These audio elements can add depth to your practice and promote relaxation.

9. Inspirational Readings: A Thoughtful Start
Many yogis like to begin their practice with a short reading or intention-setting. Have a book of inspirational quotes or a journal nearby to help you set the tone for your session.

10. Sacred Ritual: Mindfulness Moments
Create a sacred ritual before you start your practice, like lighting a candle or taking a few moments for quiet reflection. This ritual signifies the transition from your daily life to your dedicated yoga time.

11. Uninterrupted Time: Prioritize Your Practice
Lastly, prioritize uninterrupted time for your practice. Communicate with those around you to ensure you won't be disturbed during your session. This allows you to fully immerse yourself in the experience.

Preparing your space is a powerful act of self-care and intention-setting. It sends a message to your subconscious that your practice is valuable and sacred. With a thoughtfully prepared space, you'll find it easier to focus, release stress, and connect deeply with your yoga journey. So, take the time to create your yoga sanctuary, and you'll reap the rich rewards it offers to your body, mind, and spirit.

Choosing the Right Equipment

Your Toolkit for Successful Yoga Practice
Selecting the right yoga equipment is crucial for a successful practice. Whether you're a beginner or an experienced yogi, having the appropriate tools can enhance your experience, promote safety, and provide support. Let's delve into the essentials you'll need to create your own personalized yoga toolkit.

1. Yoga Mat: The Foundation of Practice
A quality yoga mat is the cornerstone of your practice. It offers a non-slip surface, cushioning for your joints, and defines your practice space. When choosing a mat, consider its thickness, texture, and durability. Pick one that provides adequate support for your knees and a comfortable surface for poses.

2. Yoga Props: Tools for Adaptation
Yoga props, including blocks, straps, bolsters, and blankets, are invaluable for support and adaptation. Blocks aid in achieving proper alignment, straps help you reach deeper into stretches, bolsters add comfort to restorative poses, and blankets provide

cushioning or additional support. These props enable you to modify your practice based on your unique needs, especially if you have knee issues.

3. Yoga Towel: Slip-Resistant Surface

A yoga towel, typically placed on top of your mat, offers extra grip and helps absorb sweat. This is especially useful if you practice hot yoga or if your hands and feet tend to slide during your practice. Look for a towel with non-slip features.

4. Clothing: Comfort and Flexibility

Choose clothing that is both comfortable and breathable, and that allows you to move freely. Whether you prefer loose-fitting or form-fitting attire, make sure it's non-restrictive and moisture-wicking to keep you cool and comfortable during your practice.

5. Yoga Blocks: Stability and Alignment

Yoga blocks are versatile tools used to modify poses and maintain stability. They can assist in alignment, balance, and provide support for your hands, feet, or hips. Opt for blocks made of durable, lightweight materials.

6. Yoga Straps: Enhanced Flexibility

Straps are great for improving flexibility, deepening stretches, and achieving proper alignment. They're especially beneficial for individuals with limited range of motion or those recovering from knee injuries. Look for straps with adjustable lengths.

7. Bolsters: Comfort and Relaxation
Bolsters are plush cushions that add comfort and relaxation to your practice. They're commonly used in restorative poses to support the body and encourage deep relaxation. When choosing a bolster, consider the size and firmness that suits your needs.

8. Blankets: Extra Support
Yoga blankets can provide cushioning and support for various poses. They're particularly useful for seated poses, shoulder stands, and as a blanket roll for added comfort. Look for blankets made of soft, easy-to-clean material.

9. Water Bottle: Hydration
Staying hydrated is essential during your practice. Keep a water bottle within reach to ensure you can hydrate as needed. Proper hydration aids muscle and joint function.

10. Yoga Bag: Convenience and Portability
A yoga bag or carryall can help you keep your equipment organized and easily transportable. It's especially handy if you practice yoga at different

locations. Choose one with compartments to keep your mat, props, and personal items in order.

The right yoga equipment is like a supportive friend in your practice. These tools enhance your experience, allow for adaptation, and promote safety, making your yoga journey more fulfilling and effective. Invest in high-quality equipment that aligns with your needs and preferences to create a personalized yoga toolkit. With the right gear at your side, you're well-equipped to embark on your journey to better knee health and overall well-being.

Breathing Techniques

The Vital Life Force of Your Yoga Practice
In the world of yoga, breath is considered the life force, the bridge between the physical and the spiritual. It's not just inhaling and exhaling; it's a tool for harnessing energy, reducing stress, and enhancing the effectiveness of your practice. Let's delve into the art and science of breathing techniques in yoga, a practice that can revolutionize your well-being.

1. Importance of Breath in Yoga: The Prana Connection
In yoga philosophy, breath is referred to as "prana," the vital life force that sustains us. It's not just about

supplying oxygen to the body but about using the breath to influence the flow of energy (prana) throughout the body. This concept underlines the deep significance of breath in yoga.

2. Breath Awareness: A Mind-Body Link

One of the foundational aspects of yoga is breath awareness. It means paying conscious attention to your breath, aligning your mental and physical states. As you become more aware of your breath, you can use it as a tool to manage your mind and body.

3. The Three-Part Breath: Deepening the Connection

The three-part breath, or "Dirga Pranayama," is a fundamental breathing method. It involves deep, slow breaths that fill the abdomen, chest, and upper chest sequentially. This technique not only helps to expand lung capacity but also encourages relaxation and mindfulness.

4. Ujjayi Pranayama: The Ocean Breath

Ujjayi breath is often associated with the sound of the ocean. By slightly constricting the back of the throat during inhalation and exhalation, you create a soft, hissing sound. Ujjayi breath promotes concentration and helps regulate your breath during challenging poses.

5. Nadi Shodhana: The Balancing Breath
Nadi Shodhana, or alternate nostril breathing, is a technique that balances the right and left hemispheres of the brain. It is calming and brings mental clarity. By closing off one nostril at a time during inhales and exhales, you can synchronize your breathing.

6. Kapalabhati Pranayama: The Cleansing Breath
Kapalabhati is a rapid, forceful exhalation followed by a passive inhalation. It's a cleansing breath that stimulates the abdominal organs, purifies the respiratory system, and energizes the mind and body.

7. Bhramari Pranayama: The Humming Bee Breath
Bhramari involves producing a humming sound while exhaling, akin to the buzzing of a bee. This technique is soothing and helps reduce stress and anxiety. It's particularly beneficial for calming the mind and preparing for meditation.

8. Breath in Asana: Integrating with Postures
Breath and movement are intricately linked in yoga. When performing asanas (yoga postures), your breath should guide your movement. Inhales often accompany expansion or upward movements, while

exhales are linked to contraction or downward movements.

9. The Relaxation Response: Stress Reduction

One of the most powerful benefits of yoga breathing techniques is the activation of the relaxation response. Deep, mindful breaths engage the parasympathetic nervous system, reducing stress, anxiety, and promoting a state of calm and well-being.

10. Breath as Meditation: A Journey Inward

In yoga, breath can also be a focal point for meditation. Concentrating on your breath allows you to anchor your attention and delve into a state of mindfulness and inner awareness.

The art of breathing in yoga is a profound practice that extends beyond the physical realm. It's a pathway to physical health, mental clarity, and spiritual growth. By mastering various breathing techniques, you can unlock the potential of your breath to enhance your yoga practice, reduce knee discomfort, and promote overall well-being. As you continue your yoga journey, remember that your breath is always with you, ready to guide and nurture you.

Chapter 3: Foundation Poses for Knee Health

Welcome to the heart of your journey toward healthier knees. In this chapter, we'll explore a selection of foundational yoga poses meticulously chosen to strengthen, stabilize, and nurture your knees. These poses serve as the building blocks of your practice, the bedrock upon which you'll build strength, flexibility, and resilience. Join us as we dive into the world of poses designed to support and rejuvenate your knee health.

Mountain Pose

A Steady Foundation for Knee Health

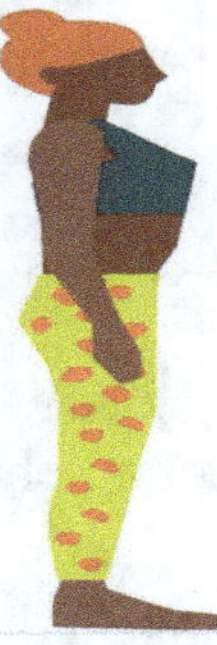

Recommended Warm-up Exercises:
Before stepping into Mountain Pose, it's vital to prepare your knees and the entire body for this foundational pose. Start with gentle joint rotations,

focusing on the ankles, knees, and hips. Dynamic stretches like leg swings can help improve circulation in the knee joints. Also, consider doing a few rounds of Sun Salutations to increase overall body flexibility and mobility.

Mountain Pose (Tadasana): Step by Step Description:

Mountain Pose may appear simple, but it forms the foundation for many yoga postures. It's a pose of alignment and stillness, where you stand tall and strong, resembling a mountain, hence the name. It may seem unassuming, but its benefits for knee health are profound.

Instructions:

1. Stand with your feet hip-width apart, toes pointing forward, and distribute your weight evenly on both feet.

2. Engage your thigh muscles to lift your kneecaps and gently tuck your tailbone.

3. Lengthen your spine, rolling your shoulders back and down, and bring your chin parallel to the ground.

4. Keep your arms relaxed by your sides with palms facing forward.

5. Breathe deeply and evenly, holding the pose with soft, yet engaged muscles.

Benefits for Knee Health:
- Strengthens Knees: Mountain Pose actively engages the muscles around your knees, helping to build strength and stability.
- Improves Alignment: It promotes proper alignment of the body, reducing the risk of knee strain and injury.
- Enhances Awareness: By focusing on posture and alignment, you become more mindful of how you carry your weight, which benefits knee health.

Alignment and Protection:
Proper alignment is crucial in Mountain Pose. Ensure your weight is evenly distributed between both feet, and your knees are not locked but slightly engaged. Soften the knees to avoid hyperextension and distribute the weight through the arches of your feet. This alignment protects the knee joints from excess stress.

Variations and Modifications:
For individuals with knee issues or different fitness levels, you can perform Mountain Pose against a wall or with a chair for support. Use the wall or chair as a reference point for alignment and balance.

Safety Precautions:
Avoid Mountain Pose if you have severe knee injuries or conditions. If you experience knee pain

during the pose, discontinue and consult a healthcare professional.

Breath and Mindfulness:
Mountain Pose provides an opportunity to focus on your breath and mindfulness. Maintain steady, deep breathing to cultivate a sense of presence and awareness.

For Beginners:
If you're new to Mountain Pose, start by practicing near a wall for support. Gradually work on your balance and alignment, and over time, you can practice without assistance.

Common Errors:
- Locking the knees: This places unnecessary strain on the knee joints. Keep your knees slightly soft.
- Poor alignment: Misalignment can lead to discomfort or pain in the knees. Ensure proper positioning and balance.

Duration and Frequency:
Hold Mountain Pose for 30 seconds to 1 minute. You can practice it daily as part of your routine to build strength and enhance knee health.

Complementary Poses:
- Chair Pose (Utkatasana): Strengthens the thighs and knee muscles.
- Tree Pose (Vrksasana): Enhances balance and stability, which benefits knee health.

Expert Insight:
As a bad knee survivor, I can attest to the power of Mountain Pose. It laid the foundation for my knee recovery journey. Its simplicity belies its impact on knee strength and overall alignment. Practicing it regularly has transformed not only my knee health but also my entire approach to well-being.

Personal Experience:
After suffering a knee injury, I was introduced to Mountain Pose as a fundamental step in my rehabilitation. The slow and steady practice allowed me to regain strength and stability in my knees. Over time, I saw a remarkable improvement, and it set the stage for my deeper exploration of yoga's benefits for knee health. This pose is the bedrock on which I rebuilt my knee's health and my overall vitality.

Warrior I and II

Fortify Your Knees with Strength and Balance

Recommended Warm-up Exercises:

Before engaging in Warrior I and II poses, it's essential to prepare your knees and the surrounding muscles. Start with leg swings and dynamic stretches to warm up your lower body. Gentle knee circles and lunges are excellent to improve mobility and circulation around the knee joints. Gradually build up to these poses by doing them as part of a sequence with a certified instructor.

Warrior I (Virabhadrasana I): Step by Step

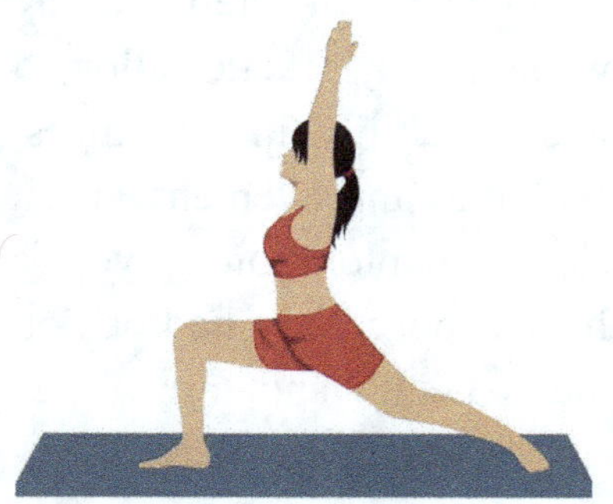

Description:

Warrior I is a powerful and grounding pose that strengthens the lower body and promotes stability. It demands strength, balance, and mindfulness.

Instructions:

1. Begin in Mountain Pose with your feet hip-width apart.

2. Step your right foot back, keeping it at a 45-degree angle, and turn your hips to face forward.

3. Inhale, raise your arms overhead, and engage your core.

4. Exhale, bend your left knee to a 90-degree angle, ensuring it aligns with your ankle.

5. Keep your back leg straight and strong, pressing the heel into the floor.

6. Gaze forward or upward, aligning your head with your biceps.

7. Hold the pose, breathing deeply, for 30 seconds to 1 minute.

8. Repeat on the other side.

Warrior II (Virabhadrasana II): Step by Step

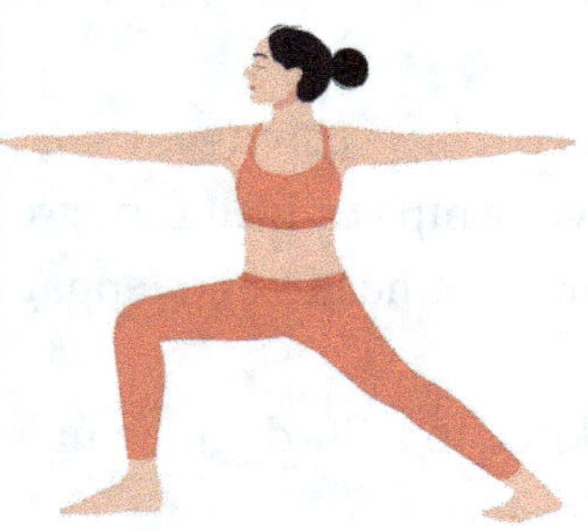

Description:
Warrior II is a dynamic pose that strengthens and stretches the legs, improving flexibility and balance. It's excellent for promoting knee stability.

Instructions:
1. Start in Mountain Pose and step your right foot back, this time keeping it parallel to the back of the mat.
2. Open your hips to face the side, and extend your arms to shoulder height, palms facing down.
3. Bend your left knee to a 90-degree angle, ensuring it aligns with your ankle.
4. Keep your back leg straight and strong, pressing the outer edge of your foot into the mat.
5. Gaze over your left hand, keeping your shoulders relaxed.
6. Hold the pose for 30 seconds to 1 minute.
7. Repeat on the other side.

Benefits for Knee Health:
- Strengthens Knees: Both Warrior I and II require strong engagement of the leg muscles, including the quadriceps, which in turn, strengthens the knee joint.
- Increases Flexibility: Warrior II, in particular, helps improve knee and hip flexibility while strengthening the surrounding muscles.
- Promotes Balance: Balancing on one leg in Warrior I and maintaining the pose in Warrior II enhances overall balance, reducing the risk of knee instability.

Alignment and Protection:
Proper alignment is crucial. Ensure your bent knee in both poses is directly above your ankle, preventing strain on the knee. In Warrior II, your back foot should be parallel to the mat's edge. Maintain a strong core to support your lower back.

Variations and Modifications:
For those with knee issues or beginners, consider using a wall or a chair for support. You can also place a yoga block under your hand in Warrior II for added balance.

Safety Precautions:

Avoid these poses if you have acute knee injuries or conditions. If you experience pain or discomfort, discontinue the pose and seek advice from a healthcare professional.

Breath and Mindfulness:
Maintain steady, deep breathing in both poses. Your breath keeps you grounded and focused, enhancing balance and concentration.

For Beginners:
Start with shorter holds in these poses and gradually increase the duration as your strength and balance improve.

Common Errors:
- Allowing the front knee to go past the ankle: This can place strain on the knee joint. Keep the knee directly above the ankle.
- Collapsing the chest or rounding the back: Maintain a strong and open chest in both poses to support the lower back and knee alignment.

Duration and Frequency:
Hold each pose for 30 seconds to 1 minute, and practice them regularly to build knee strength and improve balance.

Complementary Poses:
- Tree Pose (Vrksasana): Enhances balance and strengthens the lower body.
- Extended Triangle Pose (Utthita Trikonasana): Promotes flexibility and strengthens the legs.

Expert Insight:
As a knee survivor, I have found Warrior I and II to be pivotal in my journey to knee health. These poses foster strength, balance, and alignment while simultaneously building mental resilience. The stability they bring to the knee joints has been a game-changer in my pursuit of well-being.

Personal Experience:
Warrior I and II, when practiced mindfully and with a focus on alignment, provided a solid foundation for me. They strengthened my knees, improved flexibility, and empowered me to explore more advanced poses. Today, these poses continue to be my allies in maintaining optimal knee health.

Chair Pose (Utkatasana)

Building Knee Strength and Resilience

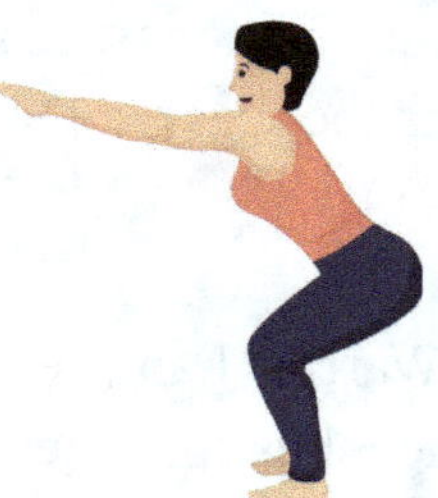

Recommended Warm-up Exercises:
Chair Pose demands strength and flexibility in the knees. To prepare, start with dynamic leg swings and knee circles. Perform deep lunges and stretches to warm up the quadriceps, hamstrings, and calves. Gradually increase your knee joint's mobility through a sequence led by a certified yoga instructor.

Description:
Chair Pose, also known as Utkatasana, is a dynamic standing pose that closely resembles sitting in an imaginary chair. This asana is an effective way to strengthen the muscles surrounding the knee joint while improving flexibility and balance.

Instructions:

1. Begin in Mountain Pose with your feet hip-width apart.

2. Inhale and raise your arms overhead, keeping them parallel to each other.

3. Exhale, bend your knees and sit back as if you're sitting in a chair. Keep your knees together and your thighs parallel to the ground.

4. Tilt your pelvis slightly to engage your core and maintain a natural arch in your lower back.

5. Ensure your weight is evenly distributed between both feet, and keep your spine straight.

6. Gaze forward and breathe deeply.

7. Maintain the posture for 30 seconds to 1 minute.

Benefits for Knee Health:

- Strengthens Knees: Chair Pose actively engages the quadriceps and hamstrings, promoting knee stability and strength.

- Increases Flexibility: While strengthening the knees, this pose also stretches and tones the calf muscles and Achilles tendons.

- Balances Weight Distribution: Chair Pose helps in balancing the weight distribution between both knees, preventing undue strain on one knee.

Alignment and Protection:

Proper alignment is crucial for knee protection. Make sure your knees do not extend past your toes.

Align them with your ankles or keep them slightly behind to protect the knee joint. Keep your core engaged and your spine straight to prevent arching the lower back.

Variations and Modifications:
For beginners or individuals with knee issues, consider practicing Chair Pose near a wall for support or by using a chair as a reference point. As you build strength, gradually work toward holding the pose for longer durations.

Safety Precautions:
Avoid Chair Pose if you have severe knee injuries or conditions. If you feel pain or discomfort in the knees, discontinue the pose and consult with a healthcare professional.

Breath and Mindfulness:
Focus on deep, even breaths during Chair Pose. Mindfulness is crucial as it helps maintain balance and proper alignment. Keep your gaze forward, and stay present in the pose.

For Beginners:
Start with shorter holds in Chair Pose and gradually increase the duration as your knee strength improves. If you have balance issues, use a wall or chair for support.

Common Errors:
- Allowing the knees to extend too far forward: This can strain the knee joint. Keep your knees aligned with your ankles or slightly behind.
- Arching the lower back: Maintain a slight tilt of the pelvis to prevent lower back strain.

Duration and Frequency:
Hold Chair Pose for 30 seconds to 1 minute. Practice it regularly, gradually increasing the duration, for optimal knee health.

Complementary Poses:
- Tree Pose (Vrksasana): Enhances balance and strengthens the lower body.
- Warrior I (Virabhadrasana I): Strengthens the knees and offers a different leg position for variety.

Expert Insight:
I've found Chair Pose to be an essential component of my routine. It's a powerful posture that has not only strengthened my knee joints but also improved my overall leg strength. Balancing in Chair Pose cultivates a sense of determination and concentration that is beneficial for overall well-being.

Personal Experience:
Chair Pose has been a game-changer in my journey to knee health. I was hesitant about practicing yoga, but Chair Pose, with its clear alignment principles and benefits for knee strength, became a vital tool in my rehabilitation. It has given me the confidence to explore and embrace other poses, strengthening my knees and improving my overall well-being.

Downward-Facing Dog (Adho Mukha Svanasana)

Elevate Your Knee Health with a Classic Pose

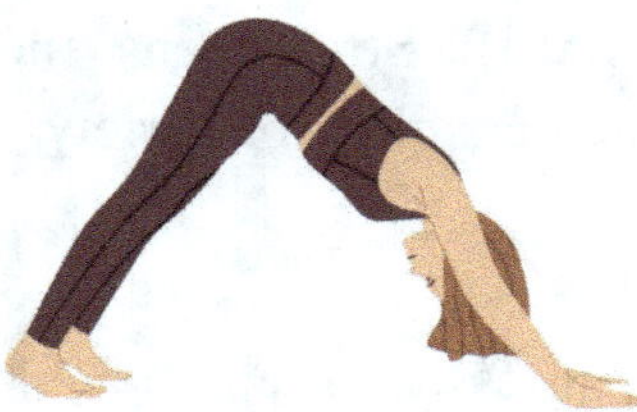

Recommended Warm-up Exercises:
Downward-Facing Dog (DFD) is a demanding pose that requires a well-prepared body, particularly the knees. Begin your warm-up with gentle knee rotations to enhance mobility. Follow this with a series of lunges to gradually awaken the quadriceps and hamstrings. Incorporate calf stretches to improve the flexibility of the lower legs. It's also a

good practice to build up to DFD through a yoga sequence under the guidance of a certified instructor.

Description:
Downward-Facing Dog is a quintessential yoga pose. It resembles an inverted "V" shape, and while it primarily targets the upper body, its benefits for knee health are profound. This asana is an all-encompassing full-body stretch that can strengthen the knees while enhancing flexibility.

Instructions:
1. Begin in a tabletop posture on your hands and knees. Your wrists should be under your shoulders, and your knees under your hips.
2. Inhale, tuck your toes under, and exhale as you lift your hips toward the ceiling.
3. Straighten your legs, but don't lock your knees. Your body should resemble an inverted "V."
4. Press your palms firmly into the ground, engage your core, and reach your hips toward the sky.
5. Keep your spine long, with your head between your arms and your gaze at your navel.
6. Press your heels toward the floor, but if your heels don't touch, it's perfectly fine. Focus on the stretch and alignment.
7. Hold the pose for 30 seconds to 1 minute, focusing on deep breaths.

Benefits for Knee Health:
- Strengthens Knees: Downward-Facing Dog is a weight-bearing pose that engages the leg muscles, particularly the quadriceps, helping to build strength in the knees.
- Increases Flexibility: This pose stretches the calf muscles and hamstrings, improving overall leg flexibility.
- Relieves Knee Pressure: DFD can reduce the load on the knees by allowing them to stretch and decompress.

Alignment and Protection:
Correct alignment is crucial to protect the knees in Downward-Facing Dog. Ensure your feet are hip-width apart and parallel. Your knees should be soft, not locked, to prevent strain. If you have tight hamstrings, you can keep a slight bend in your knees. Distribute your weight evenly between hands and feet to prevent pressure on the wrists and knees.

Variations and Modifications:
For beginners or those with knee issues, using yoga blocks under your hands can reduce the distance between the hands and the floor, making the pose more accessible. You can also practice DFD with knees slightly bent to lessen the strain on the knees.

Safety Precautions:
Avoid this pose if you have severe knee injuries or conditions. If you experience knee pain during the pose, discontinue and seek guidance from a healthcare professional.

Breath and Mindfulness:
Mindful breathing is essential in Downward-Facing Dog. As you elongate your spine and reach your hips toward the sky, take deep breaths to relax and deepen the stretch.

For Beginners:
Beginners should start with shorter holds in DFD, gradually increasing the duration as their knee strength and flexibility improve. Focus on alignment and ease into the pose to avoid overstretching.

Common Errors:
- Locking the knees: Keep your knees soft to prevent excess strain on the joint.
- Overarching the back: Maintain a long, neutral spine to protect the lower back and knees.

Duration and Frequency:
Hold Downward-Facing Dog for 30 seconds to 1 minute. It can be practiced regularly to build knee strength and improve flexibility.

Complementary Poses:
- Upward-Facing Dog (Urdhva Mukha Svanasana): Counterbalances DFD by stretching the front of the body and strengthening the upper back and knees.
- Child's Pose (Balasana): Offers a gentle stretch and relaxation for the knees, complementing the intensity of DFD.

Expert Insight:
Downward-Facing Dog has been pivotal in my journey to knee health. It's a versatile pose that not only strengthens the knees but also provides a full-body stretch. Its multifaceted benefits, from increased flexibility to improved strength, have been a game-changer in my pursuit of well-being.

Personal Experience:
When I first embarked on my path to knee recovery, Downward-Facing Dog was a challenging pose for me. With patience and regular practice, it became a cornerstone of my knee health routine. The pose's comprehensive approach to leg strength and flexibility has significantly contributed to my improved knee health and overall well-being.

Seated Forward Bend (Paschimottanasana)

Nourish Your Knees with a Soothing Stretch

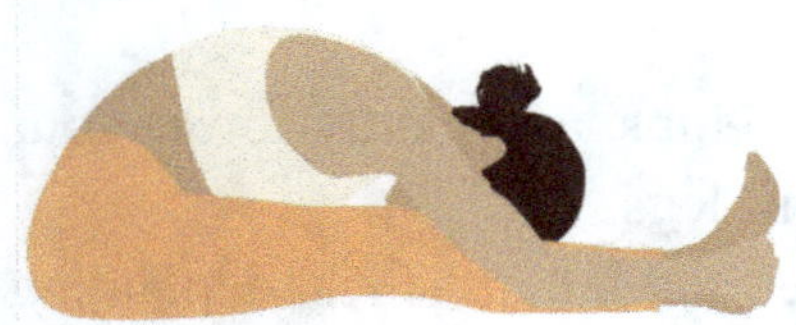

Recommended Warm-up Exercises:
To prepare your knees for Seated Forward Bend, begin with gentle knee rotations to enhance mobility. Follow this with leg swings and lunges to awaken the quadriceps, hamstrings, and calf muscles. Gradually work through a sequence of gentle stretches to ensure your knees are ready for this pose. As with any yoga practice, if you're new to it, consider guidance from a certified instructor.

Description:
Seated Forward Bend, or Paschimottanasana, is a calming seated pose that involves bending forward at the hips. While it primarily focuses on stretching the spine and hamstrings, this asana offers valuable benefits for knee health by gently strengthening and relieving tension in the knee joints.

Instructions:
1. Begin in a seated position with your legs extended in front of you.
2. Ensure your feet are flexed, toes pointing towards the ceiling.
3. Inhale, reach your arms overhead, and lengthen your spine.
4. Exhale, hinge at the hips, and gently lower your torso forward over your legs.
5. Reach for your feet, ankles, or shins, depending on your flexibility.
6. Keep your back straight and gaze forward.
7. Breathe deeply and hold the pose for 30 seconds to 1 minute.
8. Inhale as you gently raise your torso.

Benefits for Knee Health:
- Strengthens Knees: While Seated Forward Bend predominantly targets the hamstrings, the gentle engagement of the knee muscles during the pose can contribute to strengthening the knees.
- Increases Flexibility: This pose provides a deep stretch to the hamstring and calf muscles, which can aid in reducing knee discomfort and increasing flexibility.
- Relieves Knee Tension: The gentle release of tension in the knee joints, particularly when performed mindfully and with proper alignment, can contribute to knee pain relief.

Alignment and Protection:
Proper alignment is crucial for protecting the knees during Seated Forward Bend. Keep your knees extended and engage your quadriceps gently. Maintain a straight back to avoid rounding, which could strain the lower back and knees.

Variations and Modifications:
For those with knee concerns or reduced flexibility, you can use props like a yoga strap or cushion to support your forward bend. These modifications can make the pose accessible while preserving the integrity of your knee joints.

Safety Precautions:
If you have acute knee injuries or severe knee conditions, be cautious when practicing Seated Forward Bend. Avoid overstretching and discontinue if you experience knee pain.

Breath and Mindfulness:
Focus on deep, conscious breathing throughout the pose. Mindfulness is key, as it allows you to tune into your body's signals and avoid overstretching the knees.

For Beginners:

Begin with shorter holds in Seated Forward Bend to acclimate your knees and gradually progress in intensity. Ensure your breath is steady and your back is straight, preventing overstretching of the knees.

Common Errors:

- Rounding the back: Maintain a straight back to protect your knees and lower back.
- Forcing the stretch: Go only as far as your body allows without discomfort.

Duration and Frequency:

Hold Seated Forward Bend for 30 seconds to 1 minute. Regular practice can contribute to enhanced knee health. Include it in your routine, but be mindful of your body's signals.

Complementary Poses:

- Cobbler's Pose (Baddha Konasana): A gentle hip opener that can be combined with Seated Forward Bend for a well-rounded knee health routine.
- Bridge Pose (Setu Bandha Sarvangasana): Strengthens the knees and enhances overall leg muscle tone.

Expert Insight:

As someone who has navigated knee issues, Seated Forward Bend has been instrumental in my knee recovery journey. Its gentle engagement and release of knee tension, combined with enhanced flexibility, have been a boon in my pursuit of optimal knee health.

Personal Experience:

I was drawn to Seated Forward Bend for its soothing and gentle nature. Over time, this pose has played a significant role in maintaining my knee health. Its benefits extend beyond stretching and strengthening the hamstrings; it encompasses the entire knee joint. Incorporating it into my regular yoga practice has significantly contributed to my improved knee health and overall well-being.

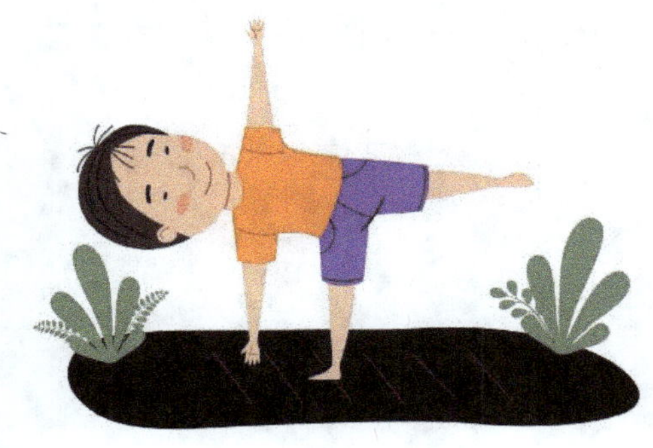

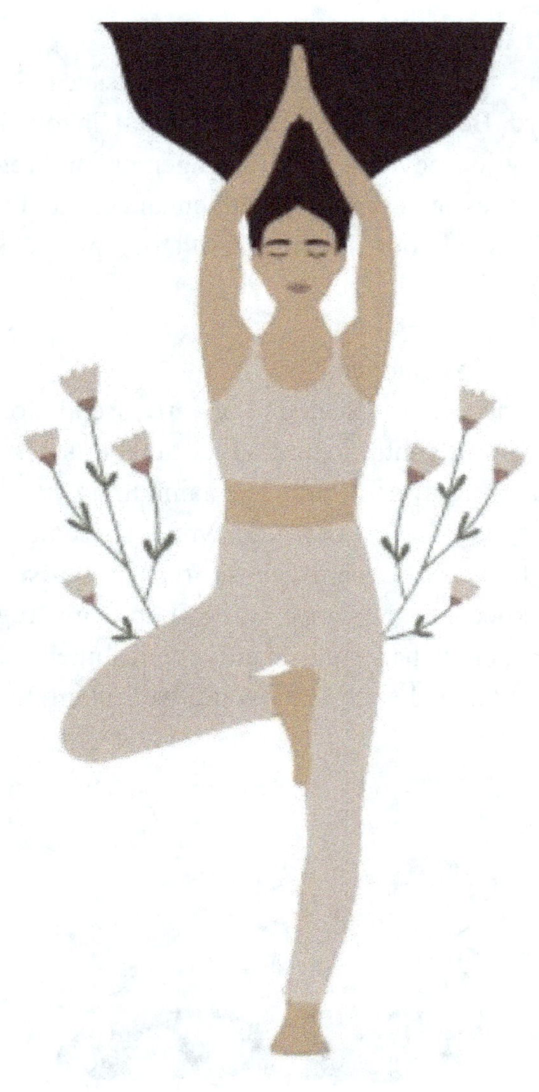

Chapter 4: Tailored Yoga Sequence

Introducing the concept of creating personalized yoga sequences to meet individual needs and goals. Its purpose is to highlight the importance of customization in yoga practice. Tailoring sequences ensures that yoga practitioners can address their unique physical, mental, and emotional requirements. By practicing a variety of sequences, individuals can experience benefits such as enhanced flexibility, strength, relaxation, and a deeper connection with their bodies and minds, ultimately fostering a more holistic approach to yoga.

Gentle Yoga For Beginners

It holds significant importance as it provides a welcoming entry point into the world of yoga. It is designed to introduce newcomers to the practice with a focus on simplicity, safety, and adaptability. This approach allows beginners to build a strong foundation, develop flexibility, and increase body awareness without the intimidation of more advanced poses. It encourages a gradual progression and instills confidence in individuals, making yoga accessible to a wider audience, including those with physical limitations or reduced fitness levels.

Bridge Pose (Setu Bandhasana) for Healthy Knees

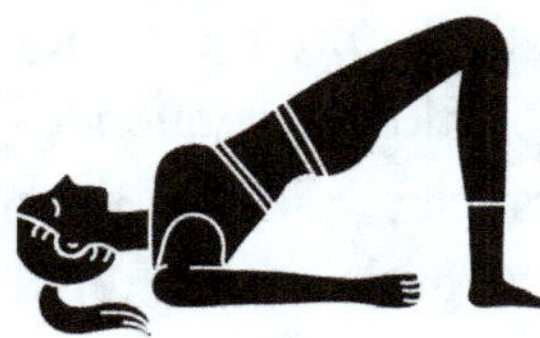

Preparing the Knees:
To prepare your knees for Bridge Pose, it's essential to engage in suitable warm-up exercises. Begin with gentle knee rotations to lubricate the joint and improve mobility. Leg lifts while lying on your back and gentle hamstring stretches can also help in warming up the knee area. Ensure your body feels loose and ready before attempting the Bridge Pose.

Bridge Pose Step-by-Step:
1. Start by lying on your back with your knees bent and feet hip-width apart. Place your arms alongside your body with palms facing down.
2. Inhale, press through your feet, and lift your hips off the mat. Keep your knees directly over your ankles, forming a straight line from shoulders to knees.

3. Engage your glutes and thighs as you lift higher. Interlace your fingers and roll your shoulders beneath your body.

4. Breathe deeply and hold the pose for several breaths.

5. To release, exhale and unclasp your hands, slowly lowering your spine back down to the mat.

Benefits for Knee Health:

Bridge Pose is an excellent yoga pose for knee health. It strengthens the muscles surrounding the knee joint, such as the quadriceps and hamstrings, providing support and stability. This pose also increases flexibility in the hip flexors and relieves stress on the knees by enhancing alignment.

Correct Body Alignment:

Maintain alignment by ensuring that your knees do not splay outwards but remain directly above your ankles. This alignment safeguards the knee joints from unnecessary strain.

Variations and Modifications:

For those with knee concerns, consider placing a block or cushion between your thighs to reduce pressure on the knees. You can also perform a supported Bridge Pose with a block beneath your sacrum. This offers a gentler version of the pose.

Safety Precautions:
Avoid Bridge Pose if you have severe knee injuries or inflammation. Always consult a healthcare professional before attempting this pose, especially if you have pre-existing knee conditions.

Breath and Mindfulness:
In Bridge Pose, focus on deep, controlled breaths. Mindfulness of your body's sensations is essential to prevent overextending the knees. Breathe into the stretch and release tension.

Beginner's Advice:
Start with a gentle lift and progress as you build strength. Avoid pushing your hips too high initially to prevent strain. Gradually extend the duration as your knees adapt.

Common Errors:
A common mistake is letting the knees splay outward, which can strain the knee joints. Keep your knees in alignment with your ankles.

Duration and Frequency:
Hold Bridge Pose for 20-30 seconds, gradually extending to 1 minute. Practice it 3-5 times a week for optimal knee health.

Complementary Poses:
To create a balanced knee health routine, follow Bridge Pose with gentle knee-to-chest stretches, Child's Pose, or Supine Hand-To-Big-Toe Pose.

While anecdotal evidence and individual experiences may attest to the benefits of Bridge Pose for knee health, always consult a healthcare professional and consider scientific studies for a more comprehensive understanding.

In my personal experience, the Bridge Pose has been instrumental in both strengthening and relieving knee discomfort. Consistent practice, along with mindfulness and proper alignment, has significantly improved my knee health. Remember, the key is to listen to your body, be patient, and practice regularly to reap the benefits. Best times for beginners to practice are in the morning or evening, 3-5 times a week, gradually increasing frequency as your knees become more resilient.

Child's Pose (Balasana) for Healthy Knees

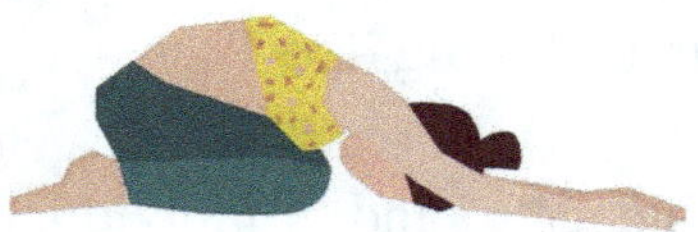

Preparing the Knees:
Before practicing Child's Pose, it's important to ensure your knees are adequately prepared. Start with gentle knee-to-chest stretches and ankle rotations to increase circulation and flexibility in the knee joint. These warm-up exercises will help your knees be more receptive to the pose.

Child's Pose Step-by-Step:
1. Begin by kneeling on the floor, big toes touching and knees spread apart.
2. Sit back on your heels and stretch your arms forward on the floor.
3. Lower your forehead to the mat, resting it on the floor.
4. Breathe deeply and hold the pose for as long as is comfortable.

Benefits for Knee Health:
Child's Pose is an excellent pose for knee health. It gently stretches the knees and promotes flexibility, relieving tension in the joint. This pose is

particularly beneficial for individuals with tight or sore knees.

Correct Body Alignment:
Ensure your knees are comfortable and that there is no strain or discomfort. Keep your toes touching and allow your knees to spread apart, but not to the point of discomfort.

Variations and Modifications:
If you experience knee discomfort, consider placing a cushion or folded blanket beneath your knees for added support. This modification reduces the pressure on the knee joint while still enjoying the benefits of the pose.

Safety Precautions:
Child's Pose is generally safe for most individuals. However, if you have a knee injury or are unable to comfortably sit back on your heels, consult a healthcare professional before attempting this pose.

Breath and Mindfulness:
Focus on your breath and relax into the pose. Deep, mindful breathing helps alleviate tension and allows you to gradually ease into the stretch, reducing strain on the knees.

Beginner's Advice:
For beginners, it's important to ease into Child's Pose and not push the stretch too far too quickly. Start with a comfortable position and gradually progress as your knee flexibility improves.

Common Errors:
A common mistake in Child's Pose is trying to force the hips to the heels, which can strain the knees. Instead, focus on a gentle stretch and let gravity do the work.

Duration and Frequency:
Maintain a Child's Pose for 30 seconds to 1 minute. This pose can be practiced daily to maintain knee flexibility and relieve discomfort.

Complementary Poses:
Child's Pose can be followed by Supine Hand-To-Big-Toe Pose (Supta Padangusthasana) to continue improving knee flexibility and overall lower body comfort.

In my personal journey, Child's Pose has been an integral part of my practice. With time, patience, and proper alignment, it has significantly improved my knee flexibility and alleviated tension. The key is to be consistent, listen to your body, and maintain mindfulness in your practice.

For beginners, the best times to practice these sequences are in the morning or evening. Initially, practice 3-5 times a week, and gradually increase the frequency as your knees become more comfortable with the poses. Remember to consult with a healthcare professional if you have existing knee issues, and always prioritize breath and mindfulness in your practice.

Supine Hand-To-Big-Toe Pose (Supta Padangusthasana) for Healthy Knees

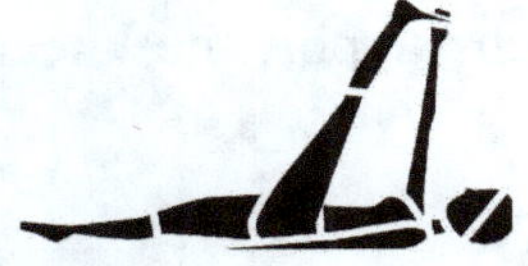

Preparing the Knees:
Before attempting Supine Hand-To-Big-Toe Pose, it's essential to ensure your knees are adequately warmed up. Start with gentle knee rotations, ankle circles, and knee-to-chest stretches. These warm-up exercises will help improve circulation and prepare the knee joints for the pose.

Supine Hand-To-Big-Toe Pose Step-by-Step:
1. Lie on your back with both legs stretched out.
2. Bend your right knee into your chest, holding it with both hands.

3. Use a strap if necessary to hold onto your right big toe.

4. Straighten your right leg upward while keeping your left leg extended on the floor.

5. Breathe deeply and hold the pose for several breaths.

6. Switch to the left leg and repeat the same steps.

Benefits for Knee Health:

Supine Hand-To-Big-Toe Pose is highly beneficial for knee health. It gently stretches the hamstrings and calf muscles, promoting flexibility and relieving knee tension. It can also help increase strength in the quadriceps, which support the knee joint.

Correct Body Alignment:

Maintain proper alignment by ensuring that the extended leg remains straight without overextending the knee. Be mindful of keeping both hips and shoulders flat on the ground.

Variations and Modifications:

If you can't reach your big toe without straining, use a yoga strap or a towel to loop around your foot. This modification allows you to experience the stretch without overtaxing the knees.

Safety Precautions:
Supine Hand-To-Big-Toe Pose is generally safe, but if you have severe knee issues or discomfort during the pose, consult a healthcare professional for guidance.

Breath and Mindfulness:
Focus on deep, mindful breathing while in this pose. Inhale as you gently stretch your leg and exhale as you relax into the stretch. This conscious breathing enhances the pose's benefits and reduces strain on the knees.

Beginner's Advice:
For beginners, it's important to start with the assistance of a strap or towel and not push the stretch too far too quickly. Gradually increase the range of motion as your knee flexibility improves.

Common Errors:
A common mistake in this pose is trying to forcefully straighten the leg. Be patient and gentle, avoiding overextension of the knee.

Duration and Frequency:
Hold each leg for 30 seconds to 1 minute, gradually increasing as your knees adapt. This pose can be practiced 3-5 times a week for optimal knee health.

Complementary Poses:
Following Supine Hand-To-Big-Toe Pose, consider practicing Child's Pose (Balasana) to further enhance knee flexibility and relieve tension.

As someone who has experienced knee discomfort, I can attest to the effectiveness of Supine Hand-To-Big-Toe Pose in promoting knee health. Consistent practice, mindfulness, and patience have significantly improved my knee flexibility and provided relief. Remember to consult with a healthcare professional, especially if you have pre-existing knee issues, and prioritize breath and mindfulness in your practice.

For beginners, the best times to practice these sequences are in the morning or evening. Initially, practice 3-5 times a week, and gradually increase the frequency as your knees become more comfortable with the poses. Your knees will thank you for the care and attention they receive through these yoga poses.

Cat-Cow Pose for Healthy Knees

Preparing the Knees:
Before you practice Cat-Cow Pose, it's important to ensure your knees are adequately prepared. Start with some gentle knee rotations to increase blood flow to the joint and warm up the surrounding muscles. Ankle circles and knee-to-chest stretches are also excellent warm-up exercises.

Cat-Cow Pose Step-by-Step:
1. Begin in a tabletop posture on your hands and knees. Check that your wrists are behind your shoulders and your knees are beneath your hips.
2. For the "Cat" portion, inhale as you arch your back, tuck your chin to your chest, and round your spine like an angry cat. Hold for a moment.

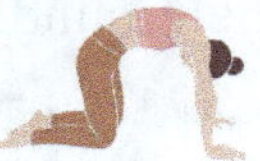

3. For the "Cow" portion, exhale as you lift your head, arch your back in the opposite direction, and look up. Your pelvis should tilt slightly upward.

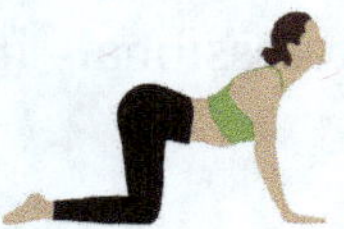

4. Flow between these two positions, inhaling into "Cat" and exhaling into "Cow."

Benefits for Knee Health:
Cat-Cow Pose is not only beneficial for spine flexibility but also for knee health. It encourages gentle knee flexion and extension, which can help maintain knee joint mobility. This pose also contributes to overall lower body circulation.

Correct Body Alignment:
Proper alignment in Cat-Cow Pose involves keeping your wrists directly under your shoulders and your knees under your hips. Maintain the natural curve of your spine in both "Cat" and "Cow" positions.

Variations and Modifications:
This pose is beginner-friendly and generally doesn't require variations or modifications for knee issues. However, if you have sensitive wrists, you can practice the pose with your forearms on the ground.

Safety Precautions:
Cat-Cow Pose is typically safe for most individuals. However, if you have severe knee pain or injuries, ensure that you do not put excessive weight on your knees and consult a healthcare professional if necessary.

Breath and Mindfulness:
Breath awareness in Cat-Cow Pose can enhance its benefits for knee health. Inhale as you round into

"Cat," and exhale as you arch into "Cow." This mindful breathing encourages relaxation and minimizes strain on the knees.

Beginner's Advice:
For beginners, it's important to start with gentle movements and not push the range of motion too far initially. Gradually increase the depth of your arches and rounds as your knees become more comfortable with the pose.

Common Errors:
One common mistake is rounding the spine too forcefully in "Cat" or over-arching it in "Cow." Maintain a gentle and controlled movement to protect your knees.

Duration and Frequency:
Flow through Cat-Cow Pose for 1-2 minutes during your yoga practice. It can be integrated into your routine every time you practice yoga for knee health.

Complementary Poses:
Following Cat-Cow Pose, consider practicing Child's Pose (Balasana) and Child's Pose (Balasana) to continue enhancing knee flexibility and lower body comfort.

Cat-Cow Pose has been an integral part of my practice. It's a gentle yet effective way to promote knee health, and with regular practice, I've noticed increased mobility and comfort in my knees. Remember to consult with a healthcare professional, especially if you have pre-existing knee issues, and prioritize breath and mindfulness in your practice.

For beginners, the best times to practice these sequences are in the morning or evening. Initially, practice 3-5 times a week, and gradually increase the frequency as your knees become more comfortable with the poses. Your knees will thank you for the care and attention they receive through these yoga poses.

Half Happy Baby Pose for Healthy Knees

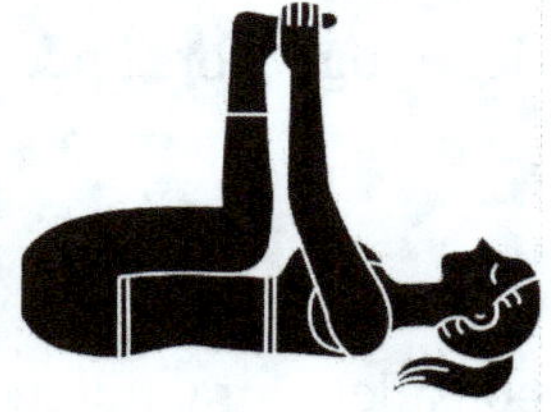

Preparing the Knees:
Before attempting Half Happy Baby Pose, it's crucial to prepare your knees. Start with gentle knee rotations and ankle circles to warm up the knee

joint. Additionally, perform knee-to-chest stretches to increase blood flow and improve knee flexibility.

Half Happy Baby Pose Step-by-Step:
1. Lie on your back with your knees bent and your feet flat on the floor.
2. Bring your right knee up to your chest.
3. Hold the outside of your right foot with your right hand, allowing your right knee to open outward.
4. Extend your left leg straight on the mat.
5. Gently pull your right knee toward the floor next to your torso, feeling a stretch in your inner thigh.
6. Breathe deeply and hold the pose for a few breaths.
7. Repeat the pose with your left leg.

Benefits for Knee Health:
Half Happy Baby Pose is excellent for knee health as it gently stretches the knee joint and inner thigh muscles. It can enhance flexibility and relieve tension in the knee area, contributing to overall knee comfort.

Correct Body Alignment:
Maintain proper alignment by keeping your extended leg straight and flat on the mat. Focus on the gentle stretch in the inner thigh without forcing your knee into an uncomfortable position.

Variations and Modifications:
For individuals with limited flexibility, consider using a yoga strap or a towel to hold onto your foot, allowing you to gently guide your knee toward the floor. This modification makes the pose accessible to a wider audience.

Safety Precautions:
Half Happy Baby Pose is generally safe, but if you have severe knee injuries or discomfort, avoid overstretching the knee or consult a healthcare professional for guidance.

Breath and Mindfulness:
Conscious breathing in Half Happy Baby Pose is vital. Inhale as you gently pull your knee toward the floor, and exhale as you relax into the stretch. This mindful approach can prevent strain on the knees.

Beginner's Advice:
For beginners, it's important to start with gentle movements and not force your knee into an uncomfortable position. Gradually increase the depth of your stretch as your knee flexibility improves.

Common Errors:
A common mistake in this pose is pulling the knee too forcefully, which can strain the knee joint. A gentle, gradual approach is key to protecting your knees.

Duration and Frequency:
Hold each leg for 30 seconds to 1 minute, gradually increasing the duration as your knees adapt. This pose can be practiced 3-5 times a week for optimal knee health.

Complementary Poses:
After Half Happy Baby Pose, consider practicing Supine Hand-To-Big-Toe Pose (Supta Padangusthasana) to continue enhancing knee flexibility and inner thigh comfort.

Half Happy Baby Pose has played a vital role in my practice. With regular practice, patience, and proper alignment, I've noticed increased knee flexibility and comfort. Remember to consult with a healthcare professional, especially if you have pre-existing knee issues, and prioritize breath and mindfulness in your practice.

For beginners, the best times to practice these sequences are in the morning or evening. Initially, practice 3-5 times a week, and gradually increase the frequency as your knees become more comfortable with the poses. Your knees will thank you for the care and attention they receive through these yoga poses.

Strengthening Sequence

A strengthening yoga sequence offers several benefits, including increased muscle tone and strength, improved stability and balance, enhanced posture, and better support for joints, including the knees. This type of sequence also boosts metabolism, helps with weight management, and can enhance overall physical resilience, making it a valuable addition to a well-rounded yoga practice.

Side Plank (Vasisthasana)

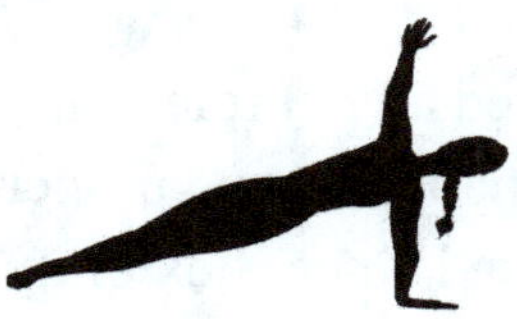

Instructions:
1. Begin in Plank Pose, with your wrists under your shoulders.
2. Shift your weight to your right hand and the outer edge of your right foot.
3. Stack your left foot on top of your right and engage your core.

4. Lift your left arm toward the ceiling.

5. Keep your body in a straight line, from head to heels.

6. Hold for several breaths, then switch sides.

Alignment and Safety Tips:

- Maintain strong core engagement to support your spine.

- For more stability, stagger your feet or keep the bottom knee on the ground.

- Avoid letting your hips sag or hiking them up too high.

Upward Facing Dog (Urdhva Mukha Svanasana)

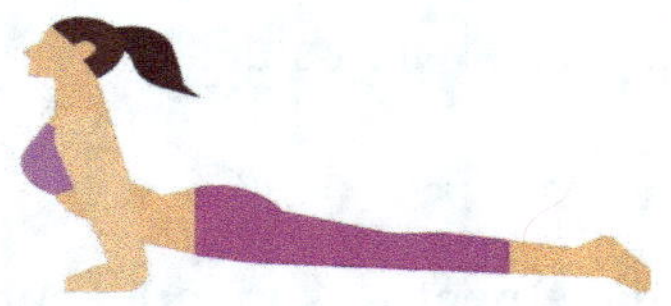

Instructions:
1. Start in Plank Pose with your palms under your shoulders.
2. Lower your body to the ground, keeping your toes pointed.
3. Inhale, press through your hands, and lift your chest and thighs off the mat.
4. Roll your shoulders back and open your heart.
5. Look forward or slightly upward.

Alignment and Safety Tips:
- Keep your wrists under your shoulders.
- Protect your lower back by using your leg muscles.
- Avoid overextending the neck; keep it in line with your spine.

Crow Pose (Bakasana)

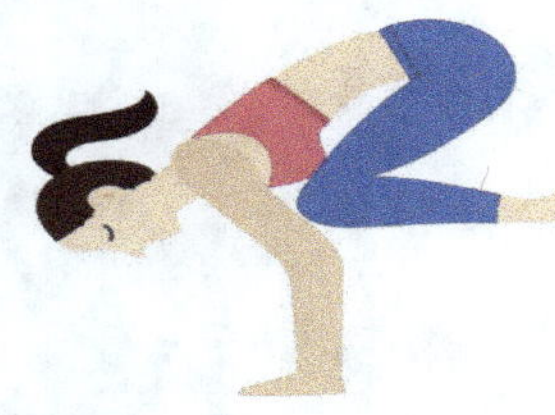

Instructions:

1. Begin in a squat position with your feet close together.

2. Place your hands on the mat, shoulder-width apart, and spread your fingers.

3. Lean forward, bend your elbows, and rest your knees on the back of your upper arms.

4. Lift your feet off the ground and shift your weight forward.

5. Balancing on your hands, engage your core.

Alignment and Safety Tips:

- Look slightly forward to maintain balance.

- To build strength, practice by lifting one foot at a time.

- Use a block under your feet or have a spotter for support.

High Lunge (Crescent Pose)

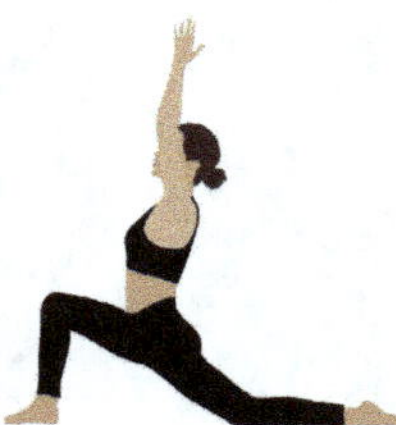

Instructions:
1. Start in Downward Facing Dog.
2. Step your right foot forward between your hands.
3. Rise up, lifting your torso and arms overhead.
4. Ensure your right knee is directly above your ankle.
5. Engage your core and reach through your fingertips.
6. Hold for several breaths, then switch sides.

Alignment and Safety Tips:
- Keep your back leg active with the heel reaching back.
- If balance is challenging, widen your stance or lower the back knee.
- Maintain a slight tuck of the tailbone to protect the lower back.

Locust Pose (Salabhasana)

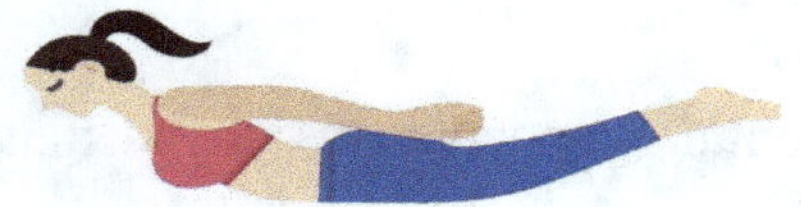

Instructions:

1. Lie on your stomach with your arms alongside your body, palms up.

2. Inhale, lift your head, chest, arms, and legs off the mat.

3. Keep your gaze down and your neck in line with your spine.

4. Engage your glutes and lower back muscles.

5. Hold the pose for a few breaths before release.

Alignment and Safety Tips:

- Avoid straining your neck; look down and keep your chin slightly tucked.

- Lift your legs by engaging your glutes, not just by bending your knees.

- If it's challenging, start by lifting one leg and then the other.

These poses are excellent for building strength. However, it's essential to practice with proper alignment and gradually progress to avoid strain or injury. Always listen to your body, and consider modifications or variations to suit your fitness level.

Flexibility and Mobility Sequence

These are fundamental aspects of yoga that contribute to overall physical well-being. Flexibility involves the lengthening and stretching of muscles, which can improve posture and reduce the risk of injury. Mobility, on the other hand, is the ability to move a joint through its full range of motion, enhancing functional movement and joint health. In yoga, a focus on both flexibility and mobility can lead to increased body awareness, reduced stiffness, and improved balance and coordination. These elements are essential for maintaining a healthy and agile body, making them a crucial component of any yoga practice.

Extended Triangle Pose (Trikonasana)

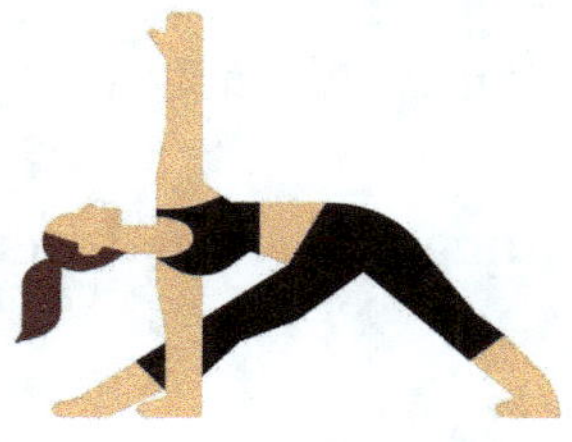

Proper Form and Technique
1. Stand with your feet wide apart, around 3-4 feet.
2. Turn your right foot out 90 degrees and your left foot slightly inwards.

3. Inhale and extend your arms out to the sides at shoulder height.

4. Exhale and reach your right hand down to your right shin, ankle, or the floor. Your left arm extends upward.

5. Keep your chest open and gaze at your left thumb.

6. Ensure your legs are straight, but don't lock your knees.

Optimal Frequency: Trikonasana can be practiced 3-5 times a week.

Complementary Exercise: Trikonasana complements strength training by enhancing flexibility and balance.

Pigeon Pose (Eka Pada Rajakapotasana):

Proper Form and Technique:

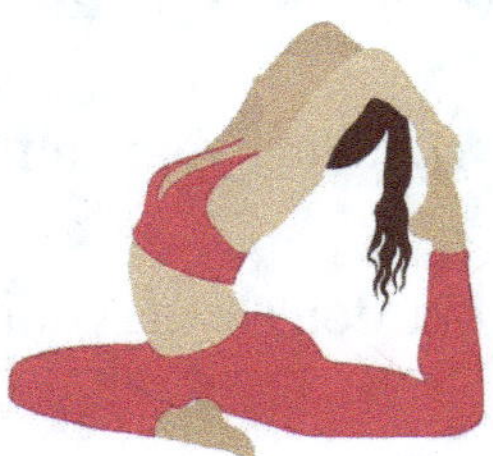

1. Start in a plank position.
2. Bring your right knee toward your right wrist and your right ankle toward your left wrist.
3. Lower your hips to the ground, extending your left leg straight back.
4. Square your hips and lower your upper body to the ground.
5. Rest on your forearms or fully extend your arms.
6. Breathe deeply and relax into the stretch.

Optimal Frequency: Practice Pigeon Pose 3-4 times a week.

Complementary Exercise: Pigeon Pose complements cardiovascular workouts by relieving tension in the hip flexors and promoting flexibility.

Butterfly Pose (Baddha Konasana):

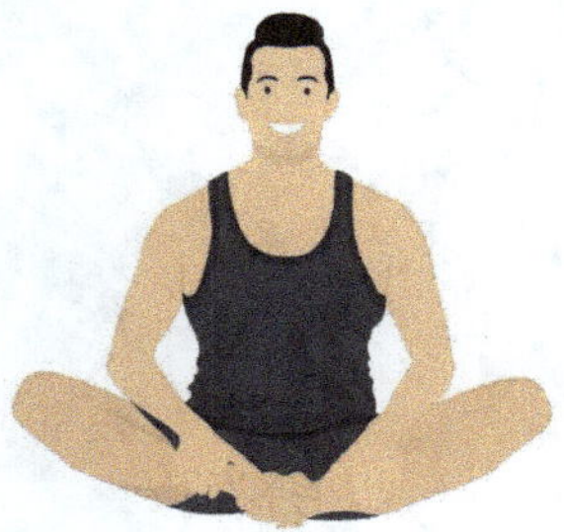

Proper Form and Technique:
1. Sit with your legs stretched out in front of you.
2. Bend your knees and bring the soles of your feet together, allowing your knees to drop to the sides.
3. Hold your feet with your hands.
4. Sit up straight and gently press your knees toward the ground.
5. Breathe deeply and relax in this seated position.

Optimal Frequency: Practice Butterfly Pose daily to improve hip flexibility.

Complementary Exercise: Butterfly Pose complements strength training by enhancing hip mobility and relieving lower back tension.

Extended Hand-To-Big-Toe Pose (Utthita Hasta Padangusthasana):

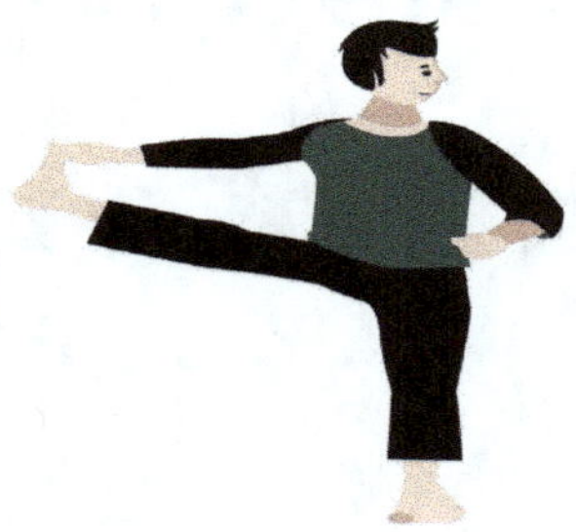

Proper Form and Technique:
1. Stand with your feet hip-width apart.
2. Shift your weight to your left leg and lift your right leg.
3. Hold your right big toe with your right hand.
4. Extend your right leg forward.
5. Keep your spine straight and gaze at a fixed point.
6. If you can't reach your toe, use a strap for assistance.

Optimal Frequency: Practice this pose 3-4 times a week.

Complementary Exercise: This pose complements agility training by improving balance and leg flexibility.

Reclining Hand-To-Big-Toe Pose (Supta Padangusthasana):

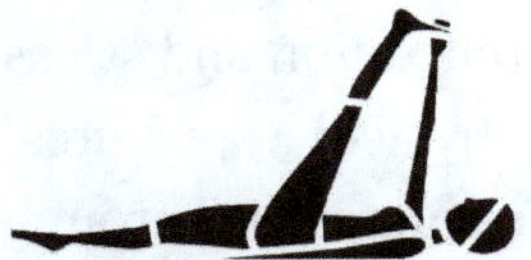

Proper Form and Technique:
1. Lie on your back with both legs stretched out.
2. Bring your right knee in close to your chest.
3. Use a strap around your right foot if necessary.
4. Extend your right leg toward the ceiling.
5. Keep your left leg extended on the floor.
6. Breathe deeply and relax into the stretch.

Optimal Frequency: Practice this pose 3-4 times a week.

Complementary Exercise: Supta Padangusthasana complements resistance training by improving hamstring and hip flexibility.

These yoga poses enhance knee flexibility and can be practiced regularly to maintain healthy joints and muscles. They complement other forms of exercise by improving overall flexibility and balance, which can help prevent injury and enhance performance.

Relaxation and Stress Relief Sequence

Yoga plays a significant role in relaxation and stress reduction by combining physical postures, controlled breathing, and mindfulness. Through yoga, individuals learn to release physical tension, regulate their breath, and calm the mind. This practice activates the body's relaxation response, reducing stress hormones and promoting a sense of inner peace. Regular yoga practice can improve stress management, reduce anxiety, and enhance overall mental and emotional well-being. It provides valuable tools to cope with the demands of daily life and find moments of serenity amidst the chaos.

Savasana (Corpse Pose):

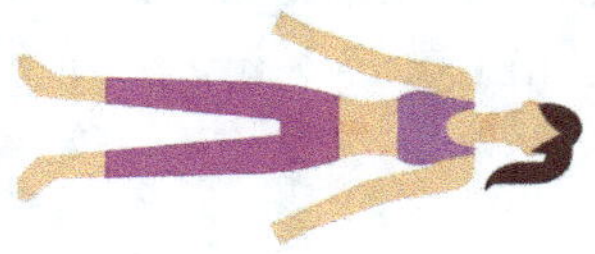

Breathwork and Meditation: As you lie in Savasana, focus on your breath. Take slow, deep breaths in and out, calming your mind. You can also incorporate a meditation technique by silently repeating a calming word or phrase with each breath.

Mindfulness: Savasana is all about being present. Allow yourself to fully relax, letting go of thoughts, and simply observe your breath and sensations.

Incorporation into Daily Life: You can practice Savasana at the end of your daily yoga session or as a standalone relaxation exercise. It's an excellent way to de-stress at the end of a long day or before bedtime.

Reclined Bound Angle Pose (Supta Baddha Konasana):

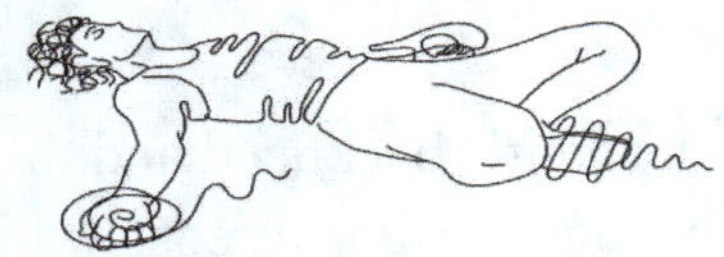

Breathwork and Meditation: Focus on your breath to release tension. Inhale deeply, feeling your belly rise, and exhale slowly, releasing any stress. You can also meditate by observing the rise and fall of your breath.

Mindfulness: As you recline in this pose, stay present with your body and sensations. Let go of any mental distractions, and embrace the feeling of release.

Incorporation into Daily Life: Practice Supta Baddha Konasana as part of a bedtime relaxation routine. This can help you relax and prepare for a good night's sleep.

Supported Bridge Pose:

Breathwork and Meditation: Use deep, rhythmic breaths to support the relaxation. You can meditate on the sensation of your heart center opening with each breath in this pose.

Mindfulness: Focus on the gentle backbend and the support of props beneath you. Let go of tension in your back and hips as you breathe deeply.

Incorporation into Daily Life: Incorporate Supported Bridge Pose into your evening routine to unwind after a busy day or before sleep.

Legs Up the Wall Pose (Viparita Karani):

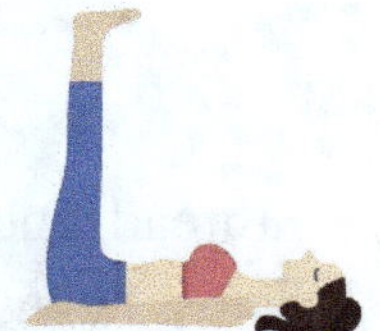

Breathwork and Meditation: Focus on your breath, inhaling and exhaling deeply. You can incorporate a meditation practice by visualizing stress leaving your body with every exhale.

Mindfulness: In Viparita Karani, embrace the feeling of relaxation and the gentle inversion. Let go of worries and distractions as you rest.

Incorporation into Daily Life: You can practice Legs Up the Wall Pose whenever you need a break from a hectic schedule. It's a wonderful pose for rejuvenation and stress relief.

Thread the Needle Pose:

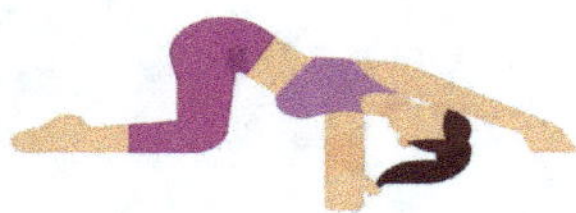

Breathwork and Meditation: As you thread one leg through the arms, take slow, deep breaths. Focus on the sensations of the stretch and meditate on the feeling of release.

Mindfulness: In Thread the Needle Pose, be present with the gentle twist and hip opening. With each breath, let rid of stress and anxiety.

Incorporation into Daily Life: This pose can be practiced as a brief break during the day, especially if you've been sitting for an extended period. It helps release lower back and hip tension.

Incorporate these sequences into your daily life by setting aside a few minutes for relaxation. They are perfect for unwinding after a long day, promoting better sleep, or taking short breaks when you need to de-stress. The importance of mindfulness in relaxation practices cannot be overstated. By being present and attentive, you can fully experience the benefits of these calming poses and flows.

Morning and Evening Routines

Morning and evening yoga routines offer distinct benefits:

Morning Routine:
- Energizes: Morning yoga awakens your body and mind, providing a gentle energy boost to start the day.
- Enhances Focus: It sets a focused and positive mindset for the day ahead.
- Improves Flexibility: Morning practice can help increase flexibility and reduce stiffness.
- Stress Reduction: Yoga reduces morning stress and anxiety, promoting emotional well-being.

Evening Routine:
- Relaxes: Evening yoga helps unwind and prepare the body for restful sleep.
- Stress Relief: It eases the tension of the day, promoting relaxation and reducing stress.
- Better Sleep: Evening practice can improve the quality of sleep and help with insomnia.
- Body Recovery: It aids in muscle recovery and can alleviate aches and pains from the day.

Both routines contribute to physical and mental well-being, but they serve different purposes in aligning with the body's natural rhythms.

Here are some morning yoga poses just for you;

Sun Salutation (Surya Namaskar):

Step by Step Instructions:

1. Begin in Mountain Pose (Tadasana).

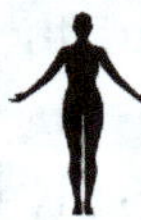

2. Inhale, raise your arms overhead, arching slightly back.

3. Exhale, bend forward into Forward Fold (Uttanasana).

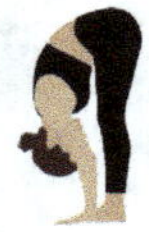

4. Inhale, step your right leg back into a lunge, and look up.

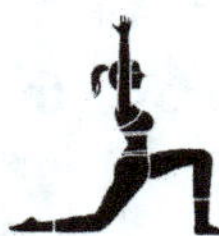

5. Exhale, step your left leg back into Plank Pose.

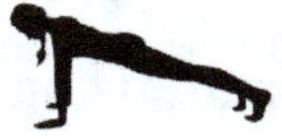

6. Lower down to the floor with your knees, chest, and chin.

7. Inhale, lift your chest into Cobra Pose (Bhujangasana).

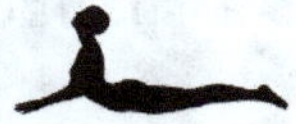

8. Exhale, lift your hips into Downward Facing Dog (Adho Mukha Svanasana).

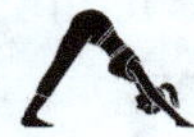

9. Inhale, step your right foot forward into a lunge.
10. Exhale, bring your left foot forward into Forward Fold.

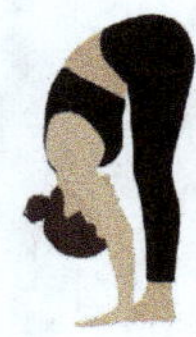

11. Inhale, come up to standing with your arms overhead.
12. Exhale, return to Mountain Pose.

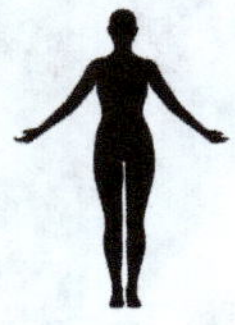

Creating a Consistent Practice Schedule: Start with 3 rounds of Sun Salutations and gradually increase. Perform it every morning at a specific time to build a habit.

Positive Impact Anecdote: Regular Sun Salutations improve flexibility, strength, and mental clarity. Practitioners often share stories of feeling more energized, balanced, and mentally prepared for the day ahead.

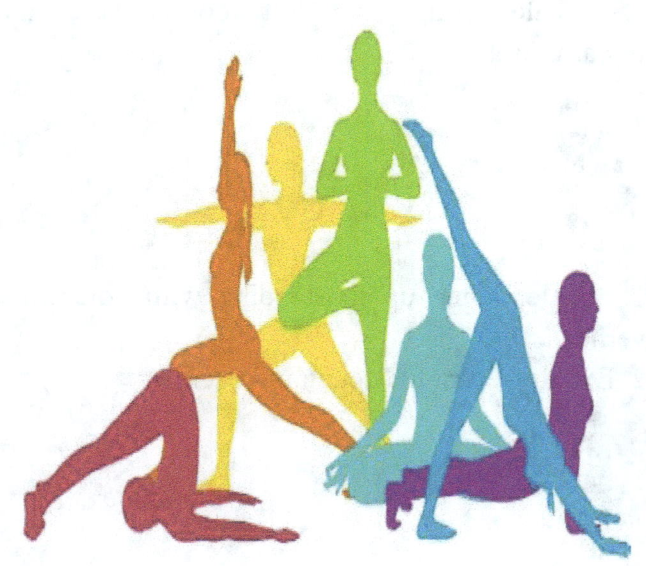

Boat Pose (Navasana):

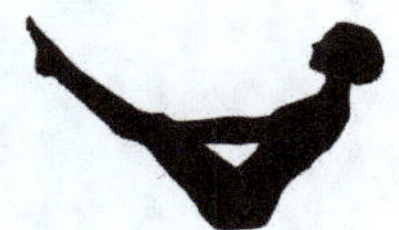

Step by Step Instructions:
1. Sit on the floor with your knees bent and feet flat.
2. Slightly lean back, leaning on your sit bones.
3. Lift your feet off the ground, keeping your legs straight.
4. Extend your arms parallel to the floor or hold onto your thighs.
5. Engage your core and balance on your sit bones.
6. Hold the pose for several breaths.

Creating a Consistent Practice Schedule: Incorporate Boat Pose into your morning routine 3 times a week. Set specific days and gradually increase the duration.

Positive Impact Anecdote: Regular practice of Boat Pose can strengthen the core muscles, enhance digestion, and boost self-confidence. Practitioners often feel a sense of empowerment and improved posture.

Camel Pose (Ustrasana):

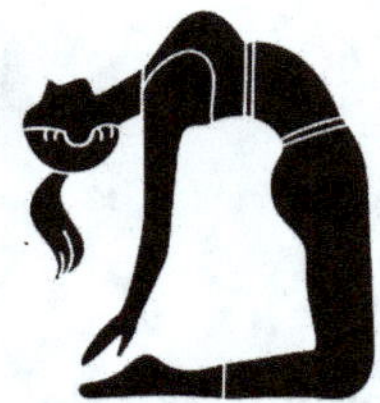

Step by Step Instructions:

1.knee and place your hands on the floor, hip-width apart.

2. Place your hands, fingers pointing downward, on your lower back.

3. Inhale, lift your chest, and gently arch backward.

4. Reach for your heels one at a time, keeping your neck in a neutral position.

5. Hold the pose for several breaths.

6. Slowly release and return to a kneeling position.

Creating a Consistent Practice Schedule: Include Camel Pose in your morning routine 2-3 times a week, with a focus on gentle backbends. Slowly increase the depth of the stretch.

Positive Impact Anecdote: Practicing Camel Pose in the morning has a profound impact on emotional well-being. Many people feel more open, compassionate, and ready to face the day's challenges with an open heart.

Twisting Chair Pose (Parivrtta Utkatasana):

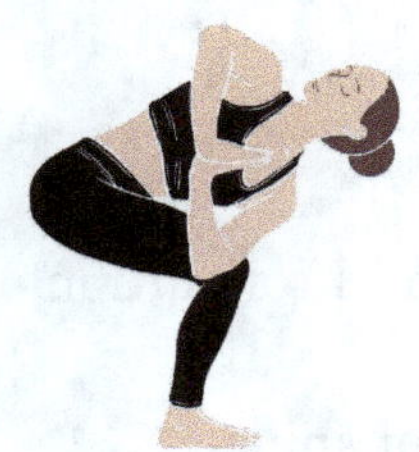

Step by Step Instructions:
1. Begin in Chair Pose (Utkatasana).
2. Bring your hands to the middle of your chest.
3. Exhale, twist to the right, hooking your left elbow outside your right thigh.
4. Keep your knees aligned and hips square.
5. Hold the twist for several breaths.
6. Inhale, return to the center, and repeat the twist on the left side.

Creating a Consistent Practice Schedule: Include Twisting Chair Pose in your morning routine 2-3 times a week. Gradually deepen the twist as you become more comfortable with the pose.

Positive Impact Anecdote: Regular twists like Parivrtta Utkatasana improve digestion and help detoxify the body. Practitioners often feel lighter and more refreshed, both physically and mentally.

Mountain Pose to Forward Fold Flow (Tadasana to Uttanasana):

Step by Step Instructions:

1. Begin in Mountain Pose (Tadasana).
2. Inhale, raise your arms overhead.
3. Exhale, hinge at your hips, and fold forward into Uttanasana.
4. Inhale, lift halfway, extending your spine.
5. Exhale, fold deeper.
6. Inhale, rise to standing with your arms overhead.
7. Exhale, return to Mountain Pose.

Creating a Consistent Practice Schedule: Start your morning with this gentle flow. Perform it daily. It's an excellent sequence to awaken your body and improve posture.

Positive Impact Anecdote: This flow enhances body awareness and posture throughout the day. Many individuals feel more aligned, graceful, and mindful after incorporating this flow into their morning routine.

These anecdotes and practice schedule suggestions highlight the transformative effects of morning yoga with specific poses, contributing to enhanced physical and emotional well-being, and setting a positive tone for the day ahead.

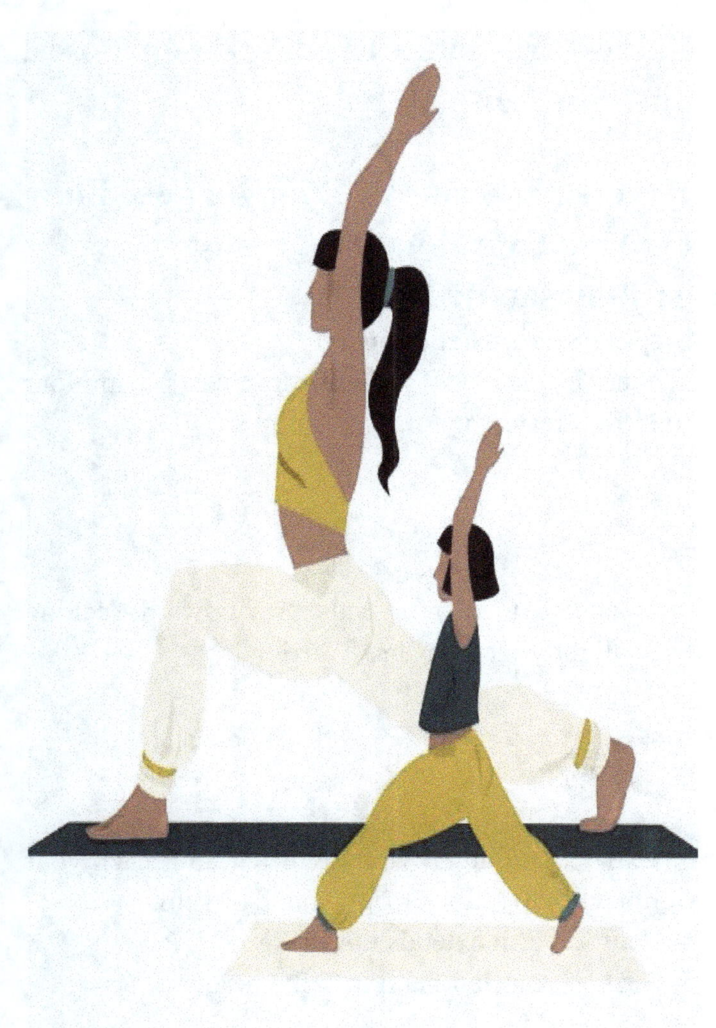

Below Are Some Evening Yoga Poses, Just For You;

Reverse Warrior to Triangle Pose Flow (Viparita Virabhadrasana to Trikonasana):

Step by Step Instructions:

1. Start in Warrior II (Virabhadrasana II) with your right foot forward.

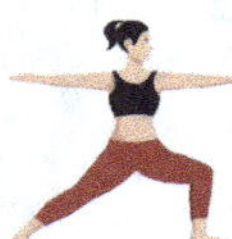

2. Inhale, extend your right arm upward, leaning back slightly into Reverse Warrior.

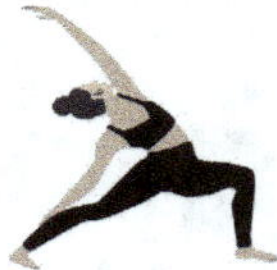

3. Exhale, straighten your right leg and reach your right hand toward your right ankle or shin.
4. Your left arm extends upward.
5. Gaze at your left hand in Trikonasana.

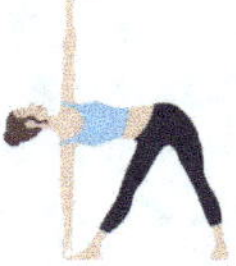

6. Repeat on the other side.

Creating a Consistent Practice Schedule: Practice this flow 3 times a week in the evening. It's excellent for knee health and improving leg strength.

Positive Impact Anecdote: Many have shared how this flow enhances knee flexibility and strengthens the legs. Practitioners often feel a sense of balance and grounding, promoting a good night's sleep.

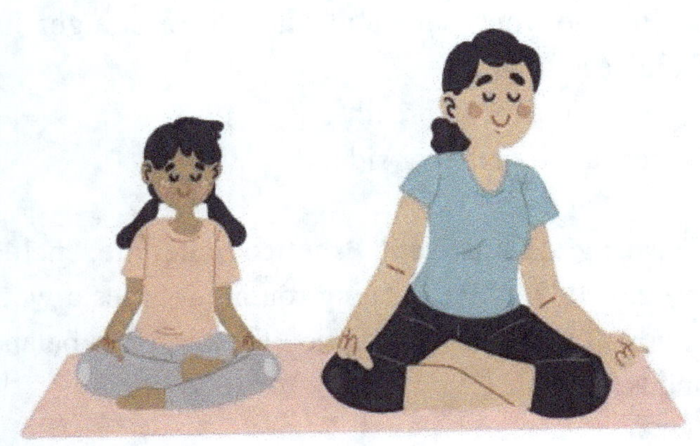

Warrior III Pose (Virabhadrasana III):

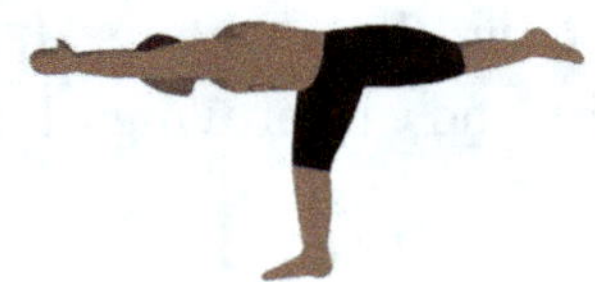

Step by Step Instructions:
1. Begin in Mountain Pose (Tadasana).
2. Transfer your weight to the right leg.
3. Inhale, lift your left leg behind you, keeping it straight.
4. Extend your arms forward, parallel to the ground.
5. Engage your core and maintain a straight line from head to heel.
6. Hold for several breaths.
7. Repeat on the other side.

Creating a Consistent Practice Schedule: Include Warrior III in your evening routine 3 times a week. Gradually extend the duration for improved balance and knee health.

Positive Impact Anecdote: Regular practice of Warrior III enhances balance, posture, and leg strength. Practitioners often share stories of improved knee stability and better sleep quality.

Tree Pose (Vrksasana):

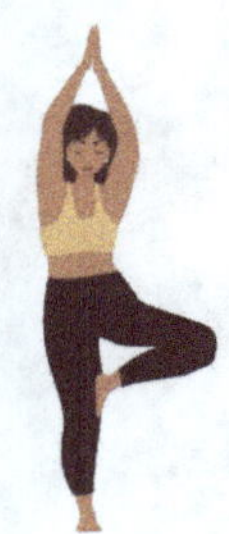

Step by Step Instructions:
1. Start in Mountain Pose (Tadasana).
2. Shift your weight to your right foot.
3. Inhale, bend your left knee, and place your left foot on your inner right thigh or calf.
4. Bring your palms to your heart center.
5. Find a focal point to aid balance.
6. Hold for several breaths.
7. Repeat on the other side.

Creating a Consistent Practice Schedule: Incorporate Tree Pose into your evening routine 3-4 times a week. Focus on balance and knee strengthening.

Positive Impact Anecdote: Practicing Tree Pose regularly improves balance, strengthens the knees, and promotes a sense of rootedness. Many individuals share stories of better knee health and an improved sense of calm before bedtime.

Savasana (Corpse Pose):

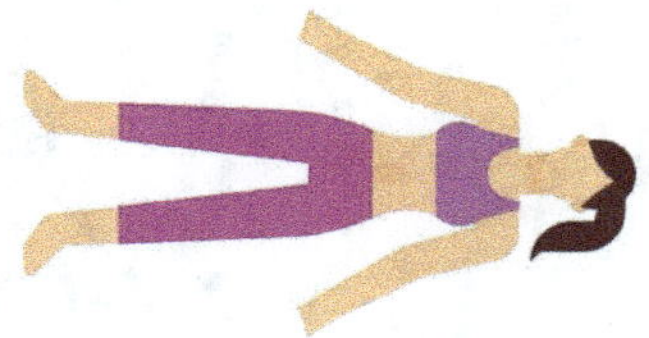

Step by Step Instructions:
1. Lie on your back with your legs extended and arms by your sides, palms facing up.
2. Close your eyes and relax your entire body.
3. Concentrate on your breath and release any tension.
4. Stay in this pose for several minutes.

Creating a Consistent Practice Schedule: End your evening practice with Savasana every day. It's a vital part of winding down and preparing for sleep.

Positive Impact Anecdote: Savasana is known for promoting relaxation and reducing stress. Practitioners often share stories of better sleep quality and a more peaceful mind.

Legs Up the Wall Pose (Viparita Karani):

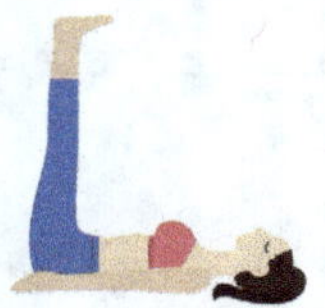

Step by Step Instructions:
1. Place your right side against the wall and sit.
2. Swing your legs up the wall as you lie down on your back.
3. Extend your legs up, resting them against the wall.
4. Relax your arms by your sides.
5. Close your eyes and concentrate on your breathing.
6. Hold this pose for a few minutes.

Creating a Consistent Practice Schedule: Incorporate Legs Up the Wall Pose into your evening routine daily. It's an excellent way to promote relaxation and knee health.

Positive Impact Anecdote: Practicing Viparita Karani regularly can reduce knee swelling and improve overall knee health. Many individuals share stories of enhanced relaxation and restful sleep.

These anecdotes and practice schedule suggestions highlight the positive impact of evening yoga with these specific poses, contributing to improved knee health and a sense of calm and balance before bedtime.

Kindly note that;

1. Yoga is a versatile and personalized practice that can be tailored to individual needs and goals.

2. Practicing a variety of yoga sequences, whether for flexibility, strength, relaxation, or knee health, offers holistic benefits to the mind and body.

3. Readers are encouraged to explore and personalize their yoga practice, adapting it to their unique requirements and schedules.

4. Yoga is not a one-size-fits-all approach; it can address specific needs and contribute to overall well-being when incorporated into daily life.

Embrace the transformative power of yoga, and remember that it's not just a physical exercise but a path to a balanced and harmonious life. Make it your own, and experience the profound positive changes it can bring to your daily existence.

Chapter 5: Modifications and Props for Healthy Knees

Now, let's delve into the world of modifications and props for maintaining and enhancing the health of your knees through yoga. Whether you're a seasoned yogi or just starting on your yoga journey, the well-being of your knees is of paramount importance. Here, we explore how to adapt your practice to protect and strengthen your knees, ensuring a safe and rewarding yoga experience. Join us as we uncover the power of props and modifications to support your knee health on the mat.

Using Props for Support

Yoga is a powerful tool for enhancing knee health, but it's essential to practice it mindfully, especially if you have knee issues or want to prevent them. One effective approach to ensure a safe and beneficial yoga practice for your knees is to incorporate props for support. These simple yet versatile tools can help you maintain proper alignment, reduce strain, and make your practice more accessible.

In this comprehensive guide, we'll explore the various props you can use and how to integrate them into your yoga routine to promote healthy knees.

Effectiveness Props For Healthy Knees:

1. Yoga Blocks:

- Yoga blocks are invaluable for providing support and stability. They can be used in standing poses, seated poses, and even during balancing sequences to make poses more achievable. For example, in Triangle Pose (Trikonasana), placing a block beneath your hand can help you reach the floor without straining your knee.

2. Yoga Straps:

- Yoga straps are excellent for increasing your reach and maintaining proper alignment. You can use them in poses like Seated Forward Bend (Paschimottanasana) to support a gentle stretch without overstretching your knee.

3. Bolsters:

- Bolsters are fantastic for providing cushioning and comfort during restorative poses. They are particularly useful in reclining poses like Reclining Hero Pose (Supta Virasana), where they can reduce the pressure on your knees and provide relaxation.

4. Blankets or Towels:

- Blankets or towels can be folded and placed under sensitive areas, such as the knees, to ease discomfort in kneeling or seated poses. They offer extra padding and support.

5. Chair:

- A sturdy chair can be a lifesaver for individuals with knee issues. It provides balance and support during standing poses, allowing you to hold the pose with less strain on your knees.

6. Wall:

- Don't underestimate the support a wall can offer. You can use it for balance, alignment, and even gentle stretches. For example, Wall Dog Pose (Adho Mukha Svanasana) allows you to stretch your calves and hamstrings without pressure on the knees.

7. Cushions or Pillows:

- Soft cushions or pillows can be placed under the knees to provide a slight elevation, relieving pressure and reducing strain during supine poses like Corpse Pose (Shavasana).

8. Inversion Aids:

- For those interested in inversions, using inversion aids like yoga slings or wall ropes can help you experience the benefits of inversions without stress on your knees.

9. Knee Pads:

- If you have specific knee issues, investing in knee pads designed for yoga can make a significant difference. They protect your knees during poses that require kneeling, like Hero Pose (Virasana).

10. Props for Balancing Poses:

- Props like balance cushions or wobble boards can assist in improving stability and strengthening the muscles surrounding your knees, which is crucial for maintaining knee health.

By incorporating these props into your yoga practice, you can tailor your routine to your specific needs and ensure a safe and enjoyable experience. Remember that the primary goal of using props is to support your knees, not to push yourself into poses that may cause discomfort or harm. Listen to your body, consult with a qualified yoga instructor or healthcare provider, and make the most of props as allies in your journey to healthier knees through yoga.

Using props for support during yoga is not a sign of weakness but a wise choice for a safer and more effective practice, leading to improved knee health and overall well-being.

Gentle Variations for Sensitive Knees

Caring for Your Joint Health

For individuals with sensitive knees, engaging in physical activities can be challenging. However, it's crucial to understand that you don't have to give up on exercise altogether. This guide explores gentle variations of exercises and activities that can help you maintain your joint health while avoiding unnecessary strain on your knees.

The Importance of Knee Health:

Knees are vital joints that support our mobility and balance. When knees are sensitive or injured, it can impact our daily lives and hinder our ability to stay active. Therefore, it's essential to prioritize knee health.

Gentle Variations of Common Exercises:

1. Low-Impact Aerobics:

- Traditional aerobic exercises like running or jumping can be harsh on sensitive knees. Instead, opt for low-impact activities such as walking, swimming, or using an elliptical machine.

- These exercises provide cardiovascular benefits without the jarring impact on your knees.

2. Yoga:

- Yoga offers a gentle way to improve flexibility and strength while also enhancing joint health.

- Focus on poses that are kind to your knees, such as child's pose, cat-cow, or seated forward bends. Always use props like yoga blocks to support your practice.

3. Strength Training:

- Muscles around your knees can be strengthened to give additional support. Opt for exercises that target the quadriceps, hamstrings, and calves.

- Leg lifts, seated leg curls, and wall squats are excellent choices. Start with low weights and gradually increase resistance.

4. Tai Chi:

- Tai Chi is a low-impact martial art that focuses on balance, flexibility, and slow, flowing movements.

- It can help reduce knee pain and improve joint stability while promoting relaxation and stress relief.

Tips for Knee Care:

1. Warm-Up and Cool Down:

   - Always start your exercise routine with a proper warm-up to prepare your joints. Gentle knee circles and leg swings can be beneficial.

   - Finish with a cool-down to ease any tension in your knees.

2. Supportive Footwear:

   - Investing in proper, supportive shoes can reduce the strain on your knees during daily activities and exercise.

3. Listen to Your Body:

   - Pay attention to how your knees feel during and after exercise. If you experience pain or discomfort, adjust your routine and consider consulting a healthcare professional.

4. Maintain a Healthy Weight:

   - Excess weight puts more strain on your knees. Achieving and maintaining a healthy weight can significantly reduce knee discomfort.

5. Use Knee Braces or Supports:

   - Depending on your specific knee sensitivity, using a knee brace or support can provide added stability during exercise.

Sensitive knees shouldn't prevent you from staying active and maintaining a healthy lifestyle. By incorporating gentle variations of exercises and following proper knee care tips, you can protect your knees, improve joint health, and continue enjoying physical activities that contribute to your overall well-being. Always consult with a healthcare professional for personalized guidance and recommendations based on your unique situation.

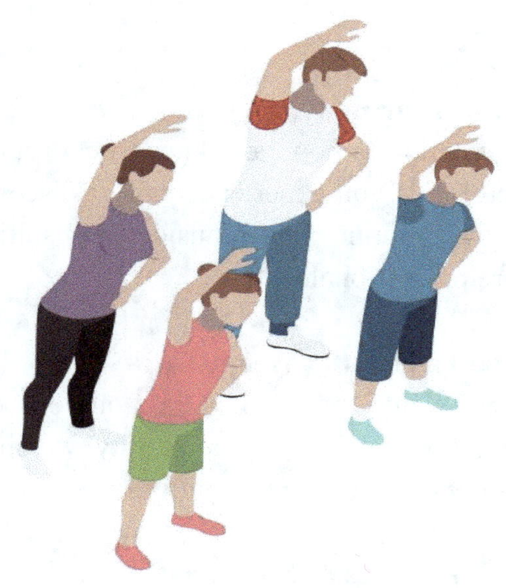

Chair Yoga Modifications

Adapting Yoga for All

Yoga is a holistic practice known for its physical, mental, and emotional benefits. However, not everyone can engage in traditional yoga poses due to physical limitations. Chair yoga offers a practical solution by modifying poses to accommodate individuals with various needs and abilities. In this guide, we will explore the world of chair yoga modifications and how they make yoga accessible to a broader audience.

What Is Chair Yoga?

Chair yoga is a gentle form of yoga that uses a chair as a prop to support yoga poses. It is ideal for people with mobility issues, seniors, office workers, or anyone seeking a less physically demanding yoga practice.

Chair Yoga Modifications:

1. Seated Poses:

   - Many classic yoga poses can be adapted for seated positions. Seated forward folds, twists, and side stretches can help improve flexibility, posture, and spinal health.

2. Chair as a Prop:

- The chair itself becomes a versatile tool. It can be used for balance support in standing poses, as a platform for seated poses, or as a support for various stretches.

3. Standing Poses:

- For those with balance issues or limited mobility, standing poses can be adapted by using the chair for support. Examples include chair-assisted tree pose and warrior poses.

4. Breathing and Meditation:

- Chair yoga emphasizes breathing and mindfulness. Seated meditation and relaxation exercises can be done comfortably in a chair, promoting inner peace and mental well-being.

5. Stretching and Flexibility:

- Chair yoga encourages gentle stretching and flexibility exercises. You can perform leg lifts, ankle circles, and arm stretches while seated, enhancing joint mobility.

6. Core Strength:

- Some core-strengthening exercises, like seated leg lifts or seated twists, can be incorporated to improve stability and support lower back health.

Benefits of Chair Yoga:

1. Accessibility:

- Chair yoga makes yoga accessible to individuals with physical limitations, injuries, or mobility challenges, ensuring that they can experience the benefits of yoga.

2. Improved Posture:

- Practicing chair yoga helps participants become more aware of their posture, reducing strain on the spine and enhancing overall posture.

3. Stress Reduction:

- Chair yoga includes mindfulness and relaxation techniques that promote stress relief and mental well-being.

4. Enhanced Mobility:

- Gentle stretches in chair yoga improve joint mobility and flexibility, making daily activities easier.

5. Community and Connection:

- Chair yoga classes provide a sense of community, helping individuals connect with others who face similar challenges.

Chair yoga modifications are a valuable addition to the world of yoga, making this ancient practice accessible to a diverse range of individuals. Whether you're recovering from an injury, dealing with limited mobility, or simply seeking a gentler yoga experience, chair yoga offers a path to improved well-being, physical health, and a sense of community. Explore chair yoga classes or use online resources to discover the benefits of this adaptable practice at your own pace.

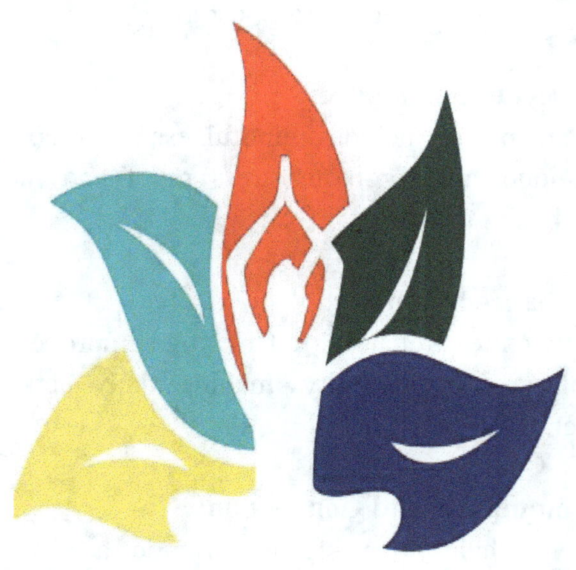

Chapter 6: Safety and Precautions

In any physical activity or practice, safety should always be a top priority. Understanding your limits, knowing when to consult a professional, and preparing for recovery are essential aspects of ensuring your well-being. In this chapter, we will delve into these critical components of maintaining safety and taking care of yourself during your journey of health and wellness.

Understanding Your Limits

Physical Limitations:

   - It's crucial to recognize and respect your body's physical limitations. Pushing oneself too hard might result in injury.

   - Listen to your body and be aware of pain, discomfort, or signs of overexertion.

Psychological Limits:

   - Mental well-being is equally important. Understand your stress and anxiety triggers, and avoid activities that may exacerbate these issues.

   - Make time for relaxation and mindfulness to maintain a healthy mental state.

The Role of Progression:

- Slow and steady progress is key to avoiding overexertion. Gradually increase the intensity and duration of your activities to allow your body to adapt.

When To Consult A Professional

Signs and Symptoms:

- Learn to recognize warning signs that may indicate the need for professional guidance. These signs can include persistent pain, joint instability, or unusual changes in physical function.

Injury Prevention:

- Seek the advice of a healthcare professional, such as a physical therapist or orthopedic specialist, to address existing injuries or prevent new ones.

- Regular check-ups can help you stay on top of your physical health.

Personalized Guidance:

- A professional can provide tailored recommendations based on your specific needs and limitations, helping you design a safer and more effective wellness program.

Preparing for Recovery

Rest and Recovery:

- Recovery is a critical aspect of any wellness routine. Make sure you allocate enough time for rest and allow your body to heal and rebuild.

Nutrition:

- Proper nutrition supports recovery by providing the necessary nutrients for tissue repair and muscle growth.

- Ensure you're consuming a well-balanced diet to aid in the recovery process.

Rehabilitation:

- If you've experienced an injury or setback, follow the prescribed rehabilitation plan provided by your healthcare professional.

- Adhering to this plan is essential for a successful recovery.

Mind-Body Connection:

- Incorporate stress-reduction techniques, such as meditation or deep breathing exercises, into your routine to support mental and emotional recovery.

Prioritizing safety and taking precautions in your health and wellness journey is paramount. Understanding your limits, seeking professional guidance when needed, and preparing for recovery are essential practices to ensure that you can continue your journey with minimal risk of injury and with a focus on holistic well-being. Remember, the key to success is to balance your ambition with responsible self-care.

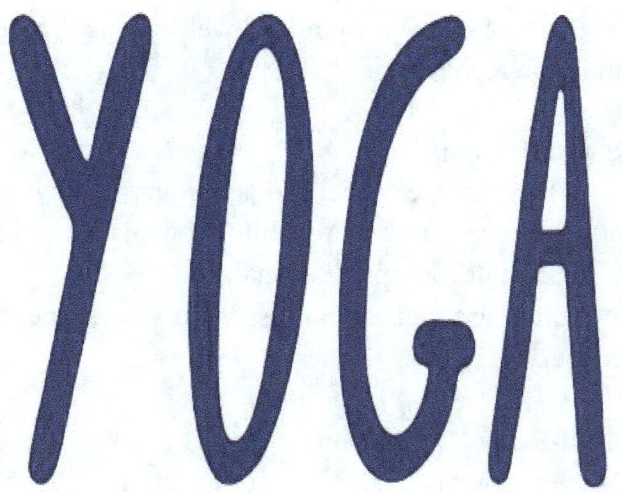

Chapter 7: Integrating Yoga into Daily Life

Yoga is more than just a physical practice; it's a way of life. In this chapter, we will explore how to seamlessly integrate yoga into your daily routine. By creating a daily practice and understanding how yoga can benefit knee health beyond the mat, you'll discover the transformative power of yoga in your everyday life.

Creating a Daily Practice

The Power of Consistency:
  - A daily yoga practice brings consistency to your life, fostering discipline, and enhancing your connection with the practice.
   - Even a short, daily session can make a significant impact over time.

Start with Breathwork:
  - Begin your day with mindful breathing exercises to center yourself and set a positive tone for the day.
   - Pranayama techniques, such as deep diaphragmatic breathing, can be integrated into your morning routine.

Morning Sun Salutations:

- A series of Sun Salutations (Surya Namaskar) is an excellent way to wake up your body, improve flexibility, and build strength.

- Customize your sequence based on your fitness level and time constraints.

Lunchtime Reset:

- Use your lunch break as an opportunity for a quick yoga session. Simple stretches and deep breathing can alleviate midday stress and refresh your mind.

Evening Relaxation:

- Wind down your day with restorative yoga poses. Practices like Yin Yoga or gentle stretching can prepare your body for a good night's sleep.

Yoga for Knee Health Beyond the Mat

Mindful Movement:

- Carry the principles of alignment and mindfulness from your yoga practice into your daily activities.

- Being aware of your posture and how you move can significantly benefit knee health.

Joint-Friendly Poses:

- Incorporate knee-friendly yoga poses and stretches into your daily life. Poses like chair pose, reclining leg stretches, and cat-cow can be done anywhere.

Supporting Knee Strength:

- Include leg lifts or knee extensions in your exercise routine to strengthen the muscles around your knees.

- Consult with a yoga instructor or physical therapist for personalized knee-strengthening routines.

Ergonomics and Alignment:

- Pay attention to your workspace and home environment. Ensure your seating and standing postures are ergonomic and knee-friendly.

- Avoid sitting for prolonged periods without taking breaks to stand or stretch.

Holistic Knee Care:
- Nutrition plays a role in knee health. A balanced diet with foods rich in anti-inflammatory properties can help reduce knee discomfort.
- Maintain a healthy weight, as excess body weight places additional stress on your knees.

Integrating yoga into your daily life is a powerful way to enhance your well-being physically, mentally, and emotionally. Creating a daily practice helps you stay consistent and disciplined, while incorporating knee-friendly yoga principles beyond the mat ensures your knees stay healthy and strong. By embracing yoga as a lifestyle, you can experience lasting improvements in your overall quality of life.

Chapter 8: Success Stories and Testimonials

In the realm of knee health and fitness, real-life transformations are the ultimate testament to the power of dedication, knowledge, and unwavering commitment. I've had the privilege of witnessing some incredible success stories throughout my career as a knee health and fitness coach, and I want to share a few of these inspiring journeys with you.

Real-life Transformations

1. Aveline Triumph Over Knee Pain

Aveline, a 45-year-old woman, came to me with chronic knee pain that had plagued her for years. She was a passionate runner, but her knees had forced her to give up her beloved sport. With a tailored plan of strengthening exercises, mobility work, and guidance on proper running form, Aveline slowly but surely began to rebuild her knee strength. Her determination was unwavering, and she started running short distances again. Over time, she not only ran a full marathon but also completed a triathlon. Aveline's transformation is a testament to the incredible resilience of the human body and the power of personalized training.

2. John's Remarkable Recovery

John, a 60-year-old gentleman, had been told by several doctors that knee replacement surgery was his only option. However, he was determined to explore alternatives. With a comprehensive program of low-impact exercises, dietary adjustments, and gentle manual therapies, John's knee pain reduced significantly. He canceled his surgery and continued to improve. Today, he enjoys hiking, gardening, and playing with his grandchildren, all without the constant agony he once endured. John's story shows that surgery isn't always the only solution, and the right guidance can make all the difference.

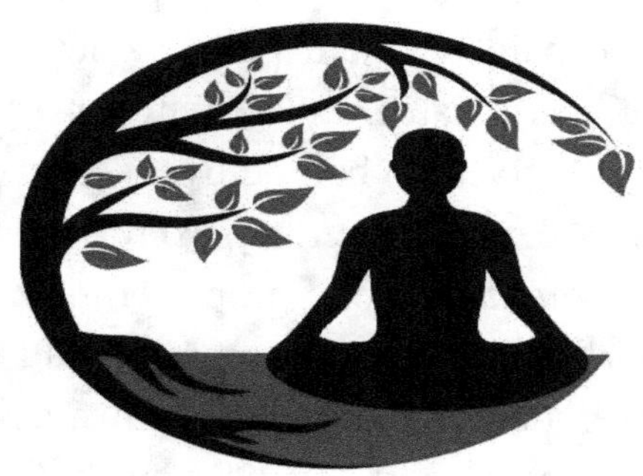

Words From Satisfied Readers

These remarkable transformations are just two examples of the countless success stories I've had the honor of being a part of. But it's not just about the physical changes; it's about the renewed sense of life, vigor, and self-confidence that these individuals gained through their journeys.

Here's what some of my happy readers had to say:

- **Jane T. (48):** "Your guidance gave me a second chance at an active life. I can now chase my kids around the park pain-free!"

- **Mark R. (55):** "I was skeptical at first, but your program turned my life around. I can't thank you enough for helping me avoid surgery."

- **Emily K. (32):** "I never thought I'd be back to running after my injury. Your holistic approach truly works, and I'm forever grateful."

As a knee health and fitness coach, these success stories are a reminder of why I do what I do. They prove that with the right knowledge, support, and determination, anyone can overcome knee pain and rediscover the joy of an active, pain-free life.

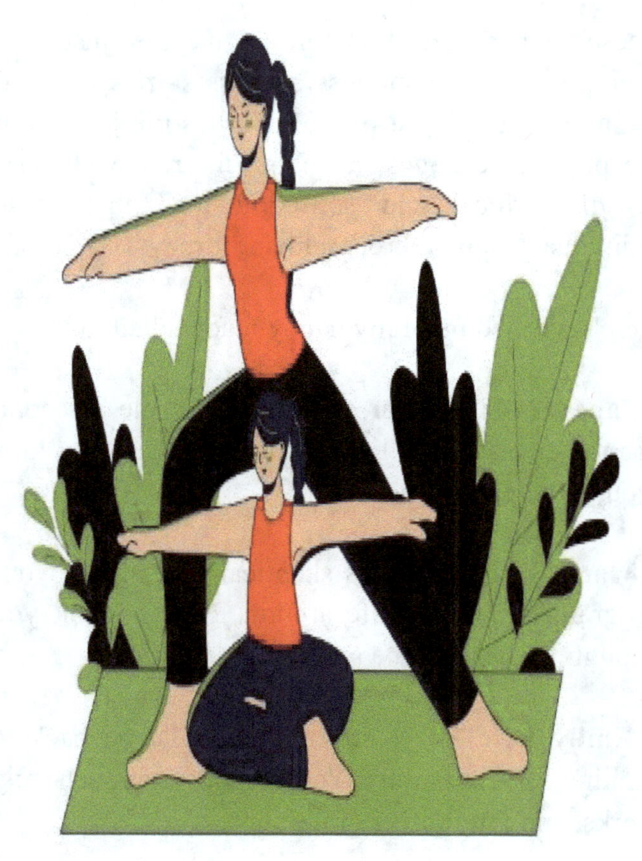

Chapter 9: Your Yoga Journey

Congratulations on embarking on your yoga journey! By now, you've likely experienced the transformative power of yoga in your life, both physically and mentally. Now, we will focus on how to maintain the progress you've made and how to embrace the yoga lifestyle fully.

Maintaining Progress

Yoga is not just a one-time endeavor; it's a lifelong journey. Whether you started your practice to improve flexibility, reduce stress, or enhance your overall well-being, consistency is key to maintaining progress. Here's how to ensure you keep reaping the benefits of yoga:

1. Regular Practice: Continue to practice yoga regularly, even if it's just a short session each day. Consistency will help maintain your flexibility, strength, and mental clarity.

2. Progressive Challenges: As you grow in your practice, challenge yourself with new poses and variations. This not only keeps things interesting but also pushes your boundaries and encourages further growth.

3. Mindful Eating: Yoga goes beyond the mat. Embrace a diet that complements your practice. Focus on whole, nutritious foods that nourish your body and mind. Take note of how eating impacts your energy levels and mood.

4. Self-Care: Self-care is an integral part of maintaining progress. Ensure you get enough sleep, manage stress, and take time for relaxation and meditation. These practices are essential for holistic well-being.

Embracing the Yoga Lifestyle

Yoga is not just a physical activity; it's a way of life. Embracing the yoga lifestyle can have a profound impact on your overall happiness and contentment. Here's how to fully integrate yoga into your daily life:

1. Mindfulness: Embrace mindfulness in every aspect of your life. Be present in each moment, whether you're at work, with family, or simply taking a walk. Mindfulness extends beyond the mat and into the world.

2. Meditation: Incorporate meditation into your daily routine. Even a few minutes of meditation can bring clarity and peace to your mind. It's a powerful tool for managing stress and enhancing focus.

3. Yogic Philosophy: Study the philosophy of yoga. Understanding concepts like the Yamas and Niyamas can help you navigate life's challenges with grace and wisdom.

4. Community: Connect with fellow yogis. Join a local yoga class or an online community. It may be quite rewarding to share your experiences and learn from others.

5. Service: Seva, or selfless service, is a core aspect of yoga. Look for methods to help your community or people in need. It's not just about physical postures but also about making the world a better place.

6. Sustainability: Embrace a sustainable lifestyle. Make eco-conscious choices that align with the principles of yoga and respect for the environment.

Your yoga journey is a lifelong adventure of self-discovery, personal growth, and well-being. By maintaining your progress and fully embracing the yoga lifestyle, you'll find that the benefits of yoga extend far beyond the mat. You'll live a more balanced, joyful, and fulfilling life, in harmony with yourself and the world around you. Continue to explore and deepen your practice, and may your yoga journey be a path to greater inner peace and enlightenment. *Namaste*.

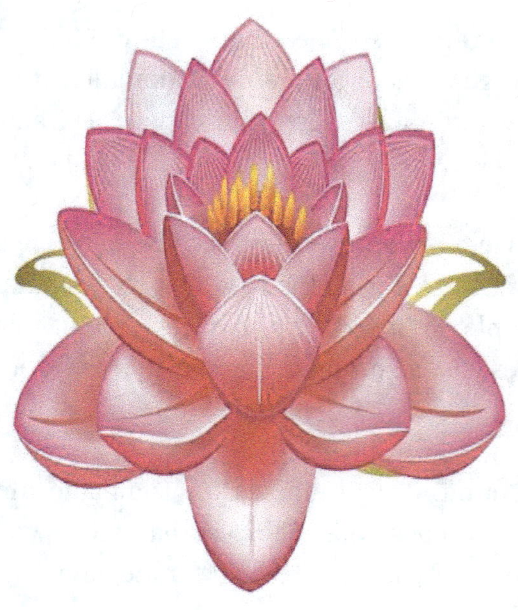

Conclusion: Your Journey Towards Healthy Knees

As we conclude our journey towards healthy knees, it's essential to reflect on the incredible strides you've made and the knowledge you've gained. Your knee health is not just a destination; it's a lifelong voyage, and you now possess the tools and understanding to navigate it successfully.

Through the chapters, we've explored the intricacies of knee anatomy, delved into the importance of proper nutrition, uncovered the secrets of effective exercise, and heard inspiring success stories of individuals who have triumphed over knee pain. You've learned to become your own advocate for knee health and have the confidence to make informed decisions.

Remember that the path to healthy knees is unique to each individual. Your journey might include moments of challenge and setbacks, but with the right mindset and guidance, you can overcome them. Whether you're an athlete striving to excel, a busy parent chasing after children, or someone simply seeking a pain-free life, the principles shared here apply to you.

The journey towards healthy knees is about more than just physical fitness; it's a holistic approach that encompasses nutrition, lifestyle, and emotional well-being. It's about understanding your body, nurturing it with care, and respecting the signals it provides.

As you continue forward, maintain a deep sense of gratitude for your body and the progress you've made. Always listen to your knees, for they have their unique language. When they whisper discomfort, it's a signal to adjust, adapt, and improve your approach. Your journey towards healthy knees is a dance, and you are the choreographer.

In your continued pursuit of knee health, remember that you are not alone. Seek support from professionals, from loved ones, and from the community of individuals who share your quest. Embrace a lifestyle that prioritizes your well-being, nourish your body with the right foods, and, most importantly, keep moving. With each step, stretch, and breath, you reaffirm your commitment to a healthier, more fulfilling life.

Your journey towards healthy knees is a testament to your strength, resilience, and determination. May it be a path filled with vitality, joy, and a profound sense of well-being. Here's to your healthy knees and the vibrant life that they enable.

"Thank you for reading, Your feedback is invaluable. If this book brightened your day or helped in any way, please share your experience by leaving a review. Your support means the world to us!"

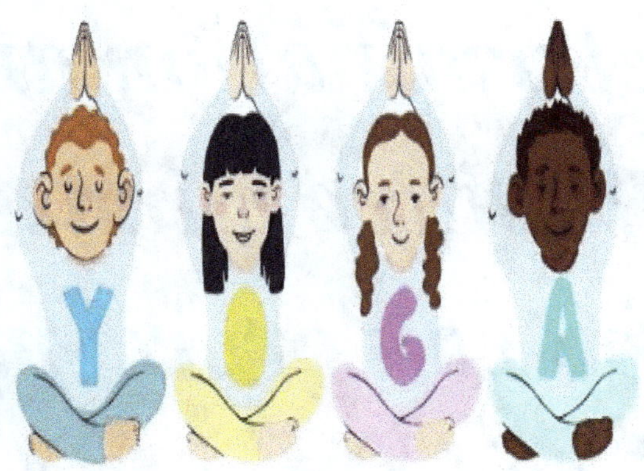

"Your knees may
be weak, but your
spirit is strong.
With
determination and
a positive mindset,
you can overcome
any obstacle."

CONGRATULATIONS ON PURCHASING YOUR NEW YOGA BOOK!

As a bonus, we're giving you access to our exclusive yoga progress tracker and FAQ section to help in improving your bad knees. This tracker will help you track your progress over time and identify areas where you need to improve. The FAQ section will answer all of your questions about yoga and bad knees.

Here's a fun way to think about it:

Imagine your knees are like two little trees. Over time, they've become weak and bent. But with regular yoga practice, you can strengthen your trees and help them grow straight and tall.

Your yoga progress tracker is like a map of your journey. It will help you see how far you've come and stay motivated to keep going. And the FAQ section is like a wise old guide who can answer all your questions and help you avoid any pitfalls.

So what are you waiting for? Start your yoga journey today!

P.S. Here's a fun fact: Did you know that yoga has been around for over 5,000 years? That's a lot of time to figure out the best way to do it, so you can be confident that you're learning from the best.

Frequently Asked Questions (FAQ)

1. Why is yoga beneficial for knee health?

- Yoga helps improve knee health by enhancing flexibility, strength, and balance. It also promotes mindfulness, which can reduce the risk of injury and enhance overall well-being.

2. Can I practice yoga for knee health if I'm a beginner?

- Absolutely! We've designed this book to cater to all levels. If you're a beginner, start with gentle poses and gradually progress. Always listen to your body and consult a yoga instructor or healthcare professional if needed.

3. What should I do if I have a knee injury or chronic knee pain?

- Consult a healthcare professional before starting any new exercise regimen. Share your concerns and seek their guidance. Yoga can often be adapted to accommodate knee issues, but it should be done under professional supervision.

4. How long should I practice yoga for healthy knees each day?

- The duration of your practice can vary. Starting with 15-30 minutes a day is great, and you can gradually increase it as your comfort and stamina improve.

5. What is the best time of day to practice yoga for knee health?

- The best time to practice is when it fits into your schedule and when you feel most comfortable. Some prefer morning yoga to start the day, while others find evening practice helps them relax.

6. Are there specific dietary recommendations for knee health?

- A well-balanced diet with foods rich in anti-inflammatory properties, such as omega-3 fatty acids, can support knee health. Consult a nutritionist for personalized advice.

7. How long will it take to see improvements in knee health through yoga?

- The timeline for improvement varies from person to person. Some may notice positive changes in a few weeks, while for others, it may take a few months. Consistency is key.

8. Can I combine other forms of exercise with yoga for knee health?

- Yes, you can incorporate low-impact exercises like swimming or cycling alongside yoga. Ensure these activities are safe for your knees and consult with a fitness professional if needed.

9. What should I do if I experience pain during yoga practice?

- Pain is not typical during yoga. If you experience pain, stop the pose immediately and consult a yoga instructor or healthcare provider to correct your form or find alternatives.

10. How can I stay motivated to continue my yoga practice for knee health?

- Set achievable goals, track your progress with our worksheets, and find a supportive community to stay motivated. Remember that consistency in practice will lead to long-term benefits.

My Yoga Progress Tracker

> "Your knees may falter, but your resilience is unwavering."

Date	Time	YOGA PRACTICE POSES AND DURATION	PAIN LEVEL BEFORE	PAIN LEVEL AFTER	NOTES AND REFLECTION
1/4/23	7.00AM	GENTLE WARM-UP (10 MIN) SEATED FORWARD BEND (5 MIN) CHILD'S POSE (5 MIN)	5/10	3/10	FELT SOME DISCOMFORT INITIALLY. IMPROVED FLEXIBILITY. VERY RELAXING.
2/4/23	6:30AM	KNEE-TO-CHEST STRETCH (7 MIN) STANDING QUADRICEPS STRETCH (5 MIN) SAVASANA (10 MIN)	6/10	4/10	FELT TIGHTNESS IN THE KNEE. FOCUSED ON FORM AND BALANCE. MIND FELT CALM AND BODY RELAXED.
6/4/23	8:30AM	MODIFIED DOWNWARD DOG (8 MIN) WARRIOR II (6 MIN) RELAXATION POSE (5 MIN)	4/10	2/10	IMPROVED RANGE OF MOTION. FELT STRONG AND STABLE. COMPLETE RELAXATION.

(EXAMPLE PAGE)

My Yoga Progress Tracker

"Your knees may falter, but your resilience is unwavering."

Date	Time	YOGA PRACTICE POSES AND DURATION	PAIN LEVEL BEFORE	PAIN LEVEL AFTER	NOTES AND REFLECTION

My Yoga Progress Tracker ❧

"Your knees may falter, but your resilience is unwavering."

Date	Time	YOGA PRACTICE POSES AND DURATION	PAIN LEVEL BEFORE	PAIN LEVEL AFTER	NOTES AND REFLECTION

My Yoga Progress Tracker

Date	Time	YOGA PRACTICE POSES AND DURATION	PAIN LEVEL BEFORE	PAIN LEVEL AFTER	NOTES AND REFLECTION

My Yoga Progress Tracker

"Your knees may falter, but your resilience is unwavering."

Date	Time	YOGA PRACTICE POSES AND DURATION	PAIN LEVEL BEFORE	PAIN LEVEL AFTER	NOTES AND REFLECTION

My Yoga Progress Tracker

"Your knees may falter, but your resilience is unwavering."

Date	Time	YOGA PRACTICE POSES AND DURATION	PAIN LEVEL BEFORE	PAIN LEVEL AFTER	NOTES AND REFLECTION

My Yoga Progress Tracker

"Your knees may falter, but your resilience is unwavering."

Date	Time	YOGA PRACTICE POSES AND DURATION	PAIN LEVEL BEFORE	PAIN LEVEL AFTER	NOTES AND REFLECTION

My Yoga Progress Tracker

Date	Time	YOGA PRACTICE POSES AND DURATION	PAIN LEVEL BEFORE	PAIN LEVEL AFTER	NOTES AND REFLECTION

My Yoga Progress Tracker

"Your knees may falter, but your resilience is unwavering."

Date	Time	YOGA PRACTICE POSES AND DURATION	PAIN LEVEL BEFORE	PAIN LEVEL AFTER	NOTES AND REFLECTION

My Yoga Progress Tracker

Date	Time	YOGA PRACTICE POSES AND DURATION	PAIN LEVEL BEFORE	PAIN LEVEL AFTER	NOTES AND REFLECTION

My Yoga Progress Tracker

"Your knees may falter, but your resilience is unwavering."

Date	Time	YOGA PRACTICE POSES AND DURATION	PAIN LEVEL BEFORE	PAIN LEVEL AFTER	NOTES AND REFLECTION

My Yoga Progress Tracker

"Your knees may falter, but your resilience is unwavering."

Date	Time	YOGA PRACTICE POSES AND DURATION	PAIN LEVEL BEFORE	PAIN LEVEL AFTER	NOTES AND REFLECTION

My Yoga Progress Tracker 🪷

Date	Time	YOGA PRACTICE POSES AND DURATION	PAIN LEVEL BEFORE	PAIN LEVEL AFTER	NOTES AND REFLECTION

My Yoga Progress Tracker

Date	Time	YOGA PRACTICE POSES AND DURATION	PAIN LEVEL BEFORE	PAIN LEVEL AFTER	NOTES AND REFLECTION

My Yoga Progress Tracker

Date	Time	YOGA PRACTICE POSES AND DURATION	PAIN LEVEL BEFORE	PAIN LEVEL AFTER	NOTES AND REFLECTION

My Yoga Progress Tracker

Date	Time	YOGA PRACTICE POSES AND DURATION	PAIN LEVEL BEFORE	PAIN LEVEL AFTER	NOTES AND REFLECTION

My Yoga Progress Tracker

"Your knees may falter, but your resilience is unwavering."

Date	Time	YOGA PRACTICE POSES AND DURATION	PAIN LEVEL BEFORE	PAIN LEVEL AFTER	NOTES AND REFLECTION

My Yoga Progress Tracker

"Your knees may falter, but your resilience is unwavering."

Date	Time	YOGA PRACTICE POSES AND DURATION	PAIN LEVEL BEFORE	PAIN LEVEL AFTER	NOTES AND REFLECTION

My Yoga Progress Tracker

Date	Time	YOGA PRACTICE POSES AND DURATION	PAIN LEVEL BEFORE	PAIN LEVEL AFTER	NOTES AND REFLECTION

My Yoga Progress Tracker

> "Your knees may falter, but your resilience is unwavering."

Date	Time	YOGA PRACTICE POSES AND DURATION	PAIN LEVEL BEFORE	PAIN LEVEL AFTER	NOTES AND REFLECTION

My Yoga Progress Tracker

Date	Time	YOGA PRACTICE POSES AND DURATION	PAIN LEVEL BEFORE	PAIN LEVEL AFTER	NOTES AND REFLECTION

My Yoga Progress Tracker

Date	Time	YOGA PRACTICE POSES AND DURATION	PAIN LEVEL BEFORE	PAIN LEVEL AFTER	NOTES AND REFLECTION

www.ingramcontent.com/pod-product-compliance
Lightning Source LLC
Chambersburg PA
CBHW070933260726
48661CB00003B/974